Mycoplasmosis in Animals:

Laboratory Diagnosis

Mycoplasmosis in Animals: Laboratory Diagnosis

EDITED BY

HOWARD W. WHITFORD

RICARDO F. ROSENBUSCH

LLOYD H. LAUERMAN

COMPILED BY THE

**Mycoplasmosis Committee
of the American Association of
Veterinary Laboratory Diagnosticians**

IOWA STATE UNIVERSITY PRESS / AMES

Ag-VetMed

SF

809

. M9 M53

1994

Howard W. Whitford, DVM, PhD, Texas Veterinary Medical Diagnostic Laboratory, College Station, TX and Diplomate, American College of Veterinary Microbiologists.

Ricardo F. Rosenbusch, DVM, MS, PhD, Veterinary Medical Research Institute, College of Veterinary Medicine, Iowa State University, Ames, IA and Diplomate, American College of Veterinary Microbiologists.

Lloyd H. Lauerman, DVM, MS, PhD, C. S. Roberts Veterinary Diagnostic Laboratory, Auburn, AL and Diplomate, American College of Veterinary Microbiologists.

© 1994 Iowa State University Press, Ames, Iowa 50014
All rights reserved

Copyright is not claimed for Chapter 3 and "Contagious Bovine Pleuropneumonia" in Chapter 5, which are in the public domain; or for Chapter 8, which was supported by Public Health Service grants RR00959 and RR00463 from the Division of Research Resources, National Institutes of Health, and funds from the Veterans Administration Research Service.

First Edition, 1994

Library of Congress Cataloging-in-Publication Data

Mycoplasmosis in animals: laboratory diagnosis/edited by Howard W. Whitford, Ricardo F. Rosenbusch, Lloyd H. Lauerman; compiled by Mycoplasmosis Committee of the American Association of Veterinary Laboratory Diagnosticians. — 1st ed.
    p.   cm.
    "Replaces Laboratory diagnosis of mycoplasmosis in food animals, published by AAVLD" — T.p. verso.
    Includes bibliographical references (p.   ) and index.
    ISBN 0-8138-2491-5
    1. Mycoplasmosis diseases — diagnosis. 2. Veterinary clinical pathology. I. Whitford, Howard W. II. Rosenbusch, Ricardo F. III. Lauerman, Lloyd H. IV. American Association of Veterinary Laboratory Diagnosticians. Mycoplasmosis Committee.
SF809.M9M53   1994
636.089′69 — dc20   93-24447

Mycoplasmosis in Animals: Laboratory Diagnosis replaces *Laboratory Diagnosis of Mycoplasmosis in Food Animals,* published by the AAVLD.

Contents

Contributors

Charles H. Armstrong, DVM, PhD (6)
29 Torchwood Court
Lafayette, IN 47905–5214

Gail H. Cassell, PhD (8)
Departments of Microbiology and
    Comparative Medicine
University of Alabama at Birmingham
Birmingham, AL 35294

Maureen Davidson, PhD (8)
Division of Comparative Medicine
c/o Animal Resources
P.O. Box 100006
University of Florida
Gainesville, FL 32610

Jerry K. Davis, DVM, PhD (8)
Department of Comparative Medicine
University of Alabama at Birmingham
Birmingham, AL 35294

Henning Ernø, DVM, DVSc
    (Addendum III)
Institute of Medical Microbiology
The Bartholin Building
University of Aarhus
DK-8000 Aarhus C
Denmark

Ginger P. Gambill, BS, MT (ASCP) (8)
Department of Microbiology
University of Alabama at Birmingham
Birmingham, AL 35294

Frederick Goll, Jr., BS, MS (3)
USDA, APHIS, NVSL
Diagnostic Bacteriology Lab
Ames, IA 50010

Donald E. Jasper, DVM, PhD (5)
Department of Clinical Pathology
School of Veterinary Medicine
University of California
Davis, CA 95616

Stanley H. Kleven, DVM, PhD (4)
University of Georgia
College of Veterinary Medicine
Department of Avian Medicine
Athens, GA 30602

Lloyd H. Lauerman, DVM, PhD (5)
C. S. Roberts Veterinary Diagnostic
    Laboratory
P.O. Box 2209
Auburn, AL 36831–2209

J. Russell Lindsey, DVM (8)
Department of Comparative Medicine
University of Alabama at Birmingham
Birmingham, AL 35294

Sonia W. Lingsweiler, BS (9)
Texas Veterinary Medical Diagnostic
    Laboratory
P.O. Drawer 3040
College Station, TX 77841

Ricardo F. Rosenbusch, DVM, PhD (1)
Veterinary Medical Research Institute
Iowa State University
Ames, IA 50011

Søren Rosendal, DVM, PhD
(7, Addendum I)
Department of Veterinary
Microbiology and Immunology
University of Guelph
Guelph, Ontario, Canada N1G 2W1

H. Louise Ruhnke, BSA, MS
(5, Addendum I)
Veterinary Laboratory Services
Ontario Ministry of Agriculture and
Food
Box 3612
Guelph, Ontario, Canada N1H 6R8

Sudhir P. Sahu, PhD (5)
USDA/APHIS
Diagnostic Virology
NVSL
P.O. Box 844
Ames, IA 50010

Howard W. Whitford, DVM, PhD
(Preface, 2, 9)
Texas Veterinary Medical Diagnostic
Laboratory
P.O. Drawer 3040
College Station, TX 77841

R. J. Yedloutschnig, DVM (5)
USDA, NVSL
Plum Island Animal Disease Center
P.O. Box 848
Greenport, NY 11944

Preface

In 1976, a special report entitled "Laboratory diagnosis of mycoplasmosis in food animals"[2] was published in the Proceedings of the Nineteenth Annual Meeting of the American Association of Veterinary Laboratory Diagnosticians (AAVLD) by its Mycoplasma Committee, chaired by Dr. Ole Stalheim. This report was copyrighted and reprinted by the AAVLD as a separate publication for several years.

In the early 1980s, revision of the 1976 report was considered by the Mycoplasmosis Committee, then chaired by Dr. C. H. Armstrong. As a two-volume textbook entitled *Methods in Mycoplasmology*[1] became available in 1983, it was decided that this reference was adequate to supplement veterinary mycoplasmology at the time. The Committee meanwhile sponsored wet-lab workshops in 1981 on swine mycoplasmas and in 1983 on ruminant mycoplasmas.

In 1987, the Committee was asked by the AAVLD Board of Governors to revise and update the original publication, which by then was outdated and in short supply. The committee agreed, and after more than 5 years of soliciting authors, reviewing papers, and making corrections, has completed the task.

We decided that this version of the publication should be expanded beyond mycoplasmosis in food animals to include companion animals (dogs, cats, horses) and laboratory rodents. The book also offers, as addenda, "Useful Protocols for Diagnosis of Animal Mycoplasmas" and "Diagnostic Index" prepared by Ms. H. L. Ruhnke and Drs. Søren Rosendal and Henning Ernø. This valuable material was originally distributed at the World Association of Veterinary Laboratory Diagnosticians mycoplasma workshop presented at Guelph, Ontario, Canada, in June 1989.

The resulting book, *Mycoplasmosis in Animals: Laboratory Diagnosis,* is especially timely as it coincides with the retirement of two "old-timers" in the field, Drs. Charles H. Armstrong and Donald E. Jasper. I personally feel fortunate that they have made, in this book, their final contribution before retirement.

The book also coincides with a change of interests on the part of Dr. Henning Ernø, who has been prominent in the field of mycoplasmosis. His collection of mycoplasma strains and antiserums has been moved to the National Collection of Type Cultures, Central Public Health Laboratory, 61 Colindale Avenue, London NW9-5HT, UK, phone 81–200–4400. This collection is perhaps the most complete repository of mycoplasma cultures and antiserums in the world.

Unfortunately, there is a paucity of mycoplasma diagnostic capability on the North American continent. To my knowledge, no veterinary diagnostic laboratory can offer a full range of service from isolation to species identification. Most laboratories are probably similar to my own, where we screen a few bovine milk samples or a few canine genital tract swabs and occasionally do tissue cultures or indirect fluorescent antibody testing on frozen sections. This seemingly low priority, along with sporadic sample submission, makes havoc for the diagnostician concerned about freshly made media, adequate controls, identification of isolates, and retention of well trained, qualified technical support.

This dilemma would be largely solved if a central laboratory, either at the state or federal level, could be established to serve the veterinary diagnostic community. However, the question of who will "foot the bill" seems to preclude establishment of such a facility at this time.

Finally, there is the problem of interpretation and even the feasibility of looking for mycoplasmas, due to the lack of applied research. What is the significance of mycoplasmas in genital tracts of dogs and cats? What, if any, are the mycoplasmas that cause problems in horses? Are mycoplasmas primary ocular pathogens in cattle, as they are in sheep? Why is ureaplasma associated with more than 10% of bovine abortions in Canada, but virtually unreported in the Southern United States? Are we not looking hard enough, or are there regional and environmental factors involved that account for the discrepancies? These and other questions are begging for answers but, for lack of controlled research studies, remain a mystery.

However, research is under way to simplify identification of mycoplasma isolates through the use of monoclonal antibodies (Dr. R. F. Rosenbusch, Iowa State University, Ames), fatty acid profiles utilizing high-resolution gas-liquid chromatography (Drs. Sang Shin and Patrick McDonough, Cornell University, Ithaca, N.Y.), and IgG Fc receptors and RNA gene probes using PCR (Dr. Lloyd Lauerman, Auburn University, Auburn, Ala.). This type of research and much more like it should one day make identification of mycoplasmas a practical and rapid procedure.

In the meantime, the Mycoplasma Committee hopes this publication will be sufficient to aid laboratory diagnosticians to offer a mycoplasma service to the veterinary community.

With great appreciation, I want to thank all of the contributors for their expertise and efforts in providing the material. In particular, for the tireless efforts of my fellow editors Drs. R. F. Rosenbusch and Lloyd Lauerman, and for the support of the Mycoplasma Committee and Board of Governors of the AAVLD, I want to extend my heartfelt gratitude. A special thank you to Ms. Ruhnke and Drs. Rosendal and Ernø for granting permission to use their material as addenda. Finally, the contributions of Ms. Sonia Lingsweiler must be recognized. She has been an invaluable asset in transferring manuscripts to computer disks, editing manuscripts for conformity, and assisting in manuscript preparation.

Howard W. Whitford

References

1. Razin S, Tully JG: 1983, Methods in mycoplasmology. Academic Press, New York.

2. Stalheim OHV, Barber TL, Blackburn BO, Frey ML, Langford EV, Livingston CW, Yedloutschnig RJ: 1976, Laboratory diagnosis of mycoplasmosis in food animals. Proc. 19th Annu Meet, Am Assoc Vet Lab Diagn.

Mycoplasmosis in Animals:

Laboratory Diagnosis

CHAPTER **1**

Biology and Taxonomy of the Mycoplasmas

R. F. ROSENBUSCH

As the smallest prokaryotes known, mycoplasmas lack several of the capabilities normally expressed by most other bacteria. Most notable among these differences is the inability to synthesize a cell wall. The absence of cell wall has been used as the primary basis for inclusion of an organism in the class Mollicutes,[3] and this feature can be documented by the demonstration that a single trilaminar membrane bounds the organism. Lack of cell wall is also the underlying reason for the "fried egg" colonial morphology that is characteristic of growth on solid media. In addition, the absence of cell wall material and cell wall–associated proteins renders mycoplasmas resistant to the action of antibiotics (such as penicillin) that interact with these proteins. Mycoplasmas have correspondingly small genomes (most have genomes that are one-sixth the size of the *Escherichia coli* genome), and their guanine plus cytosine (G + C) ratio is very low (23 to 40 mol %), so that only a part of the total genome is presumably used for expression of genetic information. As a consequence of this limited genetic potential, mycoplasmas usually require intimate association with mammalian cell surfaces and manifest complex nutritional requirements for in vitro growth. The characteristics of small size, close association to mammalian cells, and resistance to penicillin are used to design strategies for the isolation of mycoplasmas from clinical specimens (see Chapter 2).

As mentioned above, complex requirements have to be met to grow most mycoplasmas in vitro. Because of the absence of cell wall, the media used must contain adequate levels of protein to supply the necessary osmolarity. It must be prepared free of contaminants (typically introduced with poor quality laboratory water or reagents) that might inactivate enzymes on the exposed membrane of these organisms. Many mycoplasmas require an external source of sterols and fatty acids, so animal serum is generally added to the media (see Addendum I). Energy requirements of mycoplasmas are met in several ways. Glucose, either native or as a metabolizable polysaccharide, can be processed by a glycolytic pathway; arginine and active acetate can be degraded; or urea can be hydrolyzed. All of these three independent mechanisms to produce energy are coupled to a truncated respiratory system that cannot consume oxygen directly. Because of this, oxygen is neither toxic nor required for growth of mycoplasmas, making them facultative aerobes. The capability of a given mycoplasma species to use one or more of the above three methods to derive energy can be employed to aid in its characterization (Table 1.1).

The environmental resistance of mycoplasmas is of particular interest, since these organisms can be agents of infectious diseases. They can be very resistant when kept in protein-rich, moist, and cool environments. For example, *Mycoplasma dispar* has been shown to remain viable in infected lung tissue kept at 4°C for up to 14 days.[2] In contrast, many bacteria will be destroyed by autolytic activity in much shorter periods of time, under the same conditions. The significance of this environmental resistance of mycoplasmas in disease persistence has not been well documented, while other observations show that animal-to-animal transmission is involved in spread of mycoplasmal disease. In this context, biological samples suspected to contain mycoplasmas should be submitted moist and refrigerated, and processed promptly for optimum recoveries. Bacterial overgrowth is usually a much more serious problem than reduced mycoplasma survival on samples.[2] A more detailed presentation of the problems associated with collection and transport of specimens can be found in Chapter 2 of this publication and elsewhere.[1]

It has long been recognized that mycoplasmas can be highly host specific in terms of disease production. While most mycoplasmas do seem to have an absolute host specificity, others can be pathogenic in one host species and colonize other hosts without expressing pathogenicity. Some appear to have little if any host specificity but are also nonpathogenic. Since multiple mycoplasma species are often detected in samples from affected animals, it is imperative to speciate the isolates obtained from such cases. Chapter 3 covers the methodology used for identification of mycoplasmas.

Pathogenic mycoplasmas have a predilection for the respiratory, ocular, or genital mucosa and generally establish persistent superficial infections. Systemic dissemination and articular involvement can follow mucosal colonization, particularly in hosts with debilitated defenses. Some mycoplasma species have invasive properties,[4] a characteristic that is poorly

Table 1.1. Listing of mycoplasma species and basic biochemical characteristics[5]

Host	Genus and Species	Metabolic Activity[a]
PRIMATES		
Human	*Acholeplasma laidlawii*	G
	Mycoplasma buccale	A
	M. faucium	A
	M. fermentans	A,G
	M. genitalium	G
	M. hominis	A
	M. lipophilum	A
	M. orale	A
	M. penetrans	A,G
	M. pneumoniae	G
	M. primatum	A
	M. salivarium	A
	M. spermatophilum	A
	Ureaplasma urealyticum	U
Nonhuman primate living in captivity	*A. laidlawii*	G
	M. arthritidis	A
	M. buccale	A
	M. canis	G
	M. faucium	A
	M. fermentans	A,G
	M. hominis	A
	M. lipophilum	A
	M. moatsii	A,G
	M. orale	A
	M. primatum	A
	M. salivarium	A
	Ureaplasma sp.	U
Wild or recently captured primate	*M. moatsii*	A,G
DOMESTIC ANIMALS		
Cow	*A. axanthum*	G
	A. granularum	G
	A. laidlawii	G
	A. modicum	G
	Anaeroplasma abactoclasticum	G
	An. bactoclasticum	G
	M. alkalescens	A
	M. alvi	A,G
	M. arginini	A
	M. bovigenitalium	N
	M. bovirhinis	G
	M. bovis	N
	M. bovoculi	G
	M. californicum	N
	M. canadense	A
	M. canis	G
	M. capricolum	G
	M. conjunctivae	G
	M. dispar	G
	M. equirhinis	A
	M. gallinarum	A
	M. gallisepticum	G
	M. gateae	A

Table 1.1. *(Continued)*

Host	Genus and Species	Metabolic Activity[a]
DOMESTIC ANIMALS		
	M. mycoides subsp. *mycoides*	G
	M. verecundum	N
	Ureaplasma diversum	U
Bird (domestic)	*A. axanthum*	G
	A. laidlawii	G
	M. anatis	G
	M. anseris	A
	M. cloacale	A
	M. columbinasale	A
	M. columbinum	A
	M. columborale	G
	M. gallinaceum	G
	M. gallinarum	A
	M. gallisepticum	G
	M. gallopavonis	G
	M. glycophilum	G
	M. iners	A
	M. iowae	A,G
	M. lipofaciens	A,G
	M. meleagridis	A
	M. pullorum	G
	M. synoviae	G
	Ureaplasma gallorale	U
	Ureaplasma sp.	U
Horse	*A. axanthum*	G
	A. equifetale	G
	A. granularum	G
	A. hippikon	G
	A. laidlawii	G
	A. modicum	G
	A. multilocale	NR
	A. oculi	G
	A. parvum	G
	M. arginini	A
	M. bovigenitalium	N
	M. equigenitalium	G
	M. equirhinis	A
	M. fastidiosum	G
	M. feliminutum	X
	M. felis	G
	M. mycoides	G
	M. pulmonis	G
	M. salivarium	A
	M. subdolum	A
Pig	*A. axanthum*	G
	A. granularum	G
	A. laidlawii	G
	A. modicum	G
	A. oculi	G
	M. arginini	A
	M. bovigenitalium	N
	M. buccale	A
	M. flocculare	X

Table 1.1. (*Continued*)

Host	Genus and Species	Metabolic Activity[a]
	M. gallinarum	A
	M. hyopharingis	A
	M. hyopneumoniae	X
	M. hyorhinis	G
	M. hyosynoviae	A
	M. iners	A
	M. mycoides subsp. *mycoides*	G
	M. salivarium	A
	M. sualvi	A,G
	Ureaplasma sp.	U
Sheep and Goat	*A. granularum*	A
	A. laidlawii	G
	A. oculi	A
	An. abactoclasticum	G
	An. bactoclasticum	G
	Asteroleplasma anaerobium	NR
	M. agalactiae	N
	M. arginini	A
	M. bovis	N
	M. capricolum	A,G
	M. conjunctivae	G
	M. mycoides subsp. *capri*	G
	M. mycoides subsp. *mycoides*	G
	M. ovipneumoniae	G
	M. putrefaciens	G
	Taxon 2D	N
	Taxon F38	G
	Taxon G	A,G
	Taxon U	A
	Taxon V	G
	Ureaplasma sp.	U
LABORATORY ANIMALS		
Guinea pig (laboratory)	*A. cavigenitalium*	NR
	A. equifetale	G
	A. laidlawii	G
	M. caviae	G
	M. cavipharyngis	NR
	M. pulmonis	G
	Bovine group 7	NR
Chinchilla	*M. canadense*	A
Hamster, Chinese (laboratory)	*M. cricetuli*	G
	M. pulmonis	G
	M. oxoniensis	G
Hamster, Syrian (laboratory)	*M. pulmonis*	G
Mouse (field)	*M. arthritidis*	A
	M. pulmonis	G
Mouse (laboratory)	*M. arthritidis*	A
	M. collis	NR
	M. muris	A

7

Table 1.1. (*Continued*)

Host	Genus and Species	Metabolic Activity[a]
LABORATORY ANIMALS		
Mouse (laboratory)	*M. neurolyticum*	G
	M. pulmonis	G
Rabbit (laboratory)	*A. laidlawii*	G
	M. pulmonis	G
Rat (field)	*A. laidlawii*	G
Rat (laboratory)	*M. arthritidis*	A
	M. collis	NR
	M. pulmonis	G
SMALL DOMESTIC ANIMALS		
Cat	*A. laidlawii*	G
	M. arginini	A
	M. feliminutum	X
	M. felis	G
	M. gateae	A
	Ureaplasma sp.	U
Dog	*A. laidlawii*	G
	M. arginini	A
	M. bovigenitalium	N
	M. canis	G
	M. cynos	G
	M. edwardii	G
	M. feliminutum	X
	M. gateae	A
	M. maculosum	A
	M. molare	G
	M. opalescens	A
	M. spumans	A
	Ureaplasma sp.	U
WILD AND ZOO-MAINTAINED ANIMALS		
Bird (pigeon)	*M. columbinasale*	A
	M. columbinum	A
	M. columborale	G
Camel	*A. oculi*	G
Chamois	*M. conjunctivae*	G
Fish (tench)	*M. mobile*	G
Giraffe	*A. laidlawii*	G
Ground squirrel	*M. citelli*	G
Hedgehog	*A. laidlawii*	G
Lion	*M. leocaptivus*	G
	M. leopharyngis	NR
	M. simbae	NR
Llama	*M. bovis*	N

Table 1.1. (*Continued*)

Host	Genus and Species	Metabolic Activity[a]
Mouflon	*A. laidlawii*	G
Puma	*M. felifaucium*	A
Raccoon dog	*M. edwardii* *Ureaplasma* sp.	G U
Seal	*M. phocacerebrale* *M. phocarhinis* *M. phocidae*	A NR A
Shrew	*M. edwardii*	G
Tortoise	*M. testudinus*	G

[a]A = arginine utilized with media alkalinization; G = glucose utilized with media acidification; N = arginine, glucose or urea not utilized; U = urea utilized with media alklalinization; X = not definitely settled; NR = not reported.

understood at this date. These species can disseminate further and affect serosal surfaces of the thoracic, abdominal, and articular cavities of animals causing severe clinical disease. In chapters 4 through 9, specific diseases caused by mycoplasmas in various animals are covered in detail.

All mycoplasmas are included under the class Mollicutes (*mollis,* soft; *cutis,* skin), order Mycoplasmatales.[5] Subdivision into families is based on habitat, sterol requirement for growth, genome size, and oxygen tolerance. Further differentiation into genera takes into account the mechanism used by the organisms to obtain energy (i.e., glucose, arginine, or urea fermentation), as shown in Table 1.2. Mycoplasma species are defined by the above criteria, supplemented by additional biochemical properties, and by various measures of serological relatedness. Chapter 3 discusses the identification techniques that are commonly used.

Table 1.2.   Taxonomy of the Mycoplasmas[5]

Class: Mollicutes
  Order: Mycoplasmatales
    Family I: Mycoplasmataceae

    Genus I: *Mycoplasma*
      85 species described
      Genome size 600–1350 kbp (kilobase pairs)
      DNA G+C base composition 23–40 mol %
      Human and animal habitat
      Cholesterol required for growth

Table 1.2. (*Continued*)

Class: Mollicutes
  Order: Mycoplasmatales
    Family I: Mycoplasmataceae

      Genus II: *Ureaplasma*
      5 species described
      Genome size 760–1170 kbp
      DNA G+C base composition 27–30 mol %
      Urea hydrolysis
      Human and animal habitat
      Cholesterol required for growth

  Order: Entomoplasmatales
    Family I: Entomoplasmataceae

      Genus I: *Entomoplasma*
      5 species described
      Genome size 790–1140 kbp
      DNA G+C base composition 27–29 mol %
      Insect and plant habitat
      Cholesterol required for growth

      Genus II: *Mesoplasma*
      4 species described
      Genome size 870-1100 kbp
      DNA G+C base composition 27–30 mol %
      Insect and plant habitat
      No cholesterol requirement

    Family II: Spiroplasmataceae

      Genus I: *Spiroplasma*
      11 species described
      Genome size 940–2200 kbp
      DNA G+C base composition 25–30 mol %
      Insect and plant habitat
      Cholesterol required for growth

  Order III: Acholeplasmatales
    Family I: Acholeplasmataceae

      Genus I: *Acholeplasma*
      9 species described
      Genome size 1500–1650 kbp
      DNA G+C base composition 26–36 mol %
      Animals, some plants and insects as habitat
      No cholesterol requirement

  Order IV: Anaeroplasmatales
    Family: Anaeroplasmataceae

      Genus I: *Anaeroplasma*
      4 species described
      Genome size 1500–1600 kbp
      DNA G+C base composition 29–34 mol %
      Bovine/ovine rumen habitat
      Cholesterol required for growth

      Genus II: *Asteroleplasma*
      1 species described
      Genome size 1500 kbp
      DNA G+C base composition 40 mol %
      No cholesterol requirement

References

1. Clyde WA, McCormack WM: 1983, Collection and transport of specimens. In: Methods in Mycoplasmology, Vol. 1. Eds. Razin S, Tully JG., pp. 103–107. Academic Press, New York.

2. Knudtson WU, Reed DE, Daniels G: 1986, Identification of mycoplasmatales in pneumonic calf lungs. Vet Microbiol 11:79–91.

3. Subcommittee on the Taxonomy of Mollicutes: 1979, Proposal of minimal standards for descriptions of new species of the class *Mollicutes*. Int J Syst Bacteriol 29:172–180.

4. Thomas LH, Howard CJ, Parsons KR, Anger HS: 1987, Growth of *Mycoplasma bovis* in organ cultures of bovine fetal trachea and comparison with *Mycoplasma dispar.* Vet Microbiol 13:189–200.

5. Tully JG, Bové JM, Laigret F, Whitcomb RF: 1993, Revised taxonomy of the class *Mollicutes*: Proposed elevation of a monophyletic cluster of arthropod-associated mollicutes to ordinal rank (*Entomoplasmatales* ord. nov.), with provision for familial rank to separate species with nonhelical morphology (*Entomoplasmataceae* fam. nov.) from helical species (*Spiroplasmataceae*, and emended descriptions of the order *Mycoplasmatales,* family Mycoplasmataceae. Int J Syst Bacteriol 43: 378–385.

CHAPTER 2

Isolation of Mycoplasmas from Clinical Specimens

H. W. WHITFORD

This chapter describes appropriate techniques for obtaining, transporting, and processing clinical specimens to maximize the probability of recovering mycoplasmas and/or ureaplasmas. Appropriate media and their formulations are largely discussed under the chapters dealing with the various species of animals, and in Addendum I.

Since many of the mycoplasmas/ureaplasmas are very fastidious, special care must be taken to minimize loss of viable organisms. Bacterial and fungal contamination, as well as environmental extremes resulting in excessive heat, desiccation, etc., must be avoided.

Samples from live animals are limited to body secretions and accessible sites, such as natural body openings and eyes, that are amenable to swabbing. Joint fluid aspirate, transtracheal wash, endometrial lavage or biopsy, and cystocentesis require specialized methods to obtain samples for mycoplasma isolation.

In dead animals that are in a good state of preservation, samples of affected tissue with visible lesions are preferred for culture. These tissues may be seared with a hot spatula to reduce surface contamination, then cultured as one would culture for bacterial pathogens. Alternatively, the tissue may be dipped in alcohol, flamed, and minced, macerated, or ground with appropriate mycoplasma broth medium or phosphate-buffered saline (PBS). However, tissue homogenates may release mycoplasmacidal substances. Aborted fetuses and associated membranes including placenta may be processed the same as postmortem tissues.

Swabs used to collect specimens for culture must always be placed in an appropriate transport medium such as Amies' (without charcoal) or Stuart's. Dry swabs are useless if not cultured immediately after sample collection. Three cardinal rules to follow once a sample is collected are (1) keep it moist, (2) keep it cool, and (3) move fast. Isolation of mycoplasmas is maximized if samples are placed on media within a few hours of collection. If delay of a day or more is anticipated, or if a sample needs to be preserved for future culture, it should be placed in liquid nitrogen or in an ultra-cold ($-70°C$) freezer. Dry ice, although preferable to wet ice, is less effective in preserving mycoplasmas than liquid nitrogen. We have found that transporting swabs in transport medium in liquid nitrogen semen storage tanks has been highly successful in allowing the recovery of ureaplasmas from bovine genital tract swabs. Ureaplasma transport medium is available commercially (A3B [Lyophilized] [for Ureaplasma], REMEL, Lenexa, KS).

Once received at the laboratory, the samples may be plated directly on the appropriate agar-based media (usually dispensed into 50-mm plastic disposable petri dishes to conserve media). To increase the probability of isolation, part of the sample can be plated directly while part is incubated 2–3 days in broth medium before being plated. Broth-to-broth fluid passages may also increase results. Several attempts may be necessary for recovery if dealing with low numbers or fastidious organisms. Bacterial contamination may become a problem with prolonged incubation of broth tubes.

Tissue samples may be cultured by pushing a piece of aseptically collected tissue across the surface of an agar plate. Or tissues may be homogenized as previously described and titrated using serial 10-fold dilutions in the appropriate broth media, to remove mycoplasma inhibitors inherently present in tissues. Each of the dilutions is then cultured for the presence of mycoplasmas.

Most mycoplasmas grow poorly in incubators designed for aerobic conditions, as they require lowered oxygen tension and high humidity for growth. In our laboratory, we use an incubator set at $36°C$ with a 5–10% CO_2 atmosphere that is bubbled through water to maintain high humidity. Others have suggested using candle jars, but my personal experience with this method has been very disappointing. According to Dr. C. W. Livingston, there are probably some toxic products generated by the burning candle that inhibit growth of mycoplasmas.

Once plated, mycoplasmas may appear at 48–72 hours incubation; however, they may require incubation up to 10–14 days for growth to be observed. Mycoplasma colonies are easily observed with the aid of an inverted microscope equipped with a 10× objective.

Occasionally, mycoplasmas will grow on media formulated for bacterial isolation. We have recovered *M. bovis/agalactiae* from milk samples plated on 5% bovine blood agar in the course of screening for bacterial pathogens. These isolates are usually found as relatively pure cultures and appear after 48–72 hours of incubation as tiny pinpoint colonies surrounded by a small zone of beta-hemolysis. Attempts to Gram-stain these colonies are very frustrating since the colonies sink into the agar and adhere tenaciously, resulting in absence of organisms on the stained slide. If a portion of the agar containing mycoplasma is cut out and pushed across the surface of mycoplasma agar, a "bloom" of mycoplasma along the track is observed after a day or two of incubation under optimum conditions. We have also seen this occasionally when screening canine genital tract swabs for bacterial growth.

Although not often encountered in veterinary diagnostic mycoplasmology, mycoplasma-contaminated cell cultures, tissue explant and organ cultures, and egg embryos should be mentioned briefly. Such contamination is particularly important when mycoplasma become incorporated into tissues being used for research and development activities. They are often difficult to recover, and their presence is detected only by DNA staining. Appropriate antibiotic treatment has been successfully used to eliminate mycoplasma infections in cell cultures.[1]

Reference

1. Mowles JM: 1988, The use of ciprofloxacin for the elimination of mycoplasma from natural infected cell lines. Cytotechnology 1:355–358.

CHAPTER 3

Identification of Mycoplasmas Isolated from Domestic Animals

F. GOLL, JR.

Tests to detect specific enzymatic and nutritional requirements of mycoplasmas have proven useful in their classification. They are used to differentiate mycoplasmas at the family and genus level. The requirement for sterols separates the family Mycoplasmataceae from the family Acholeplasmataceae, whereas the hydrolysis of urea differentiates the genus *Ureaplasma* from the genus *Mycoplasma*. Biochemical tests are useful at the species level to characterize an isolate and narrow the choice of specific antisera or reagents needed for the final serological identification. Speciation of mycoplasmas is based on serological tests involving membrane antigens. These tests include growth inhibition, metabolic inhibition, and immunofluorescence, which can vary in their sensitivity, specificity, and ease of performance.

Preliminary Procedures

Pure Cultures

A pure mycoplasma culture is essential before any biochemical study can be performed. Picking single colonies has been used to obtain pure cultures, but mixed species of mycoplasmas can exist as clumps on agar or in broth. The recommended procedure[43] is to clone three times by gentle filtration of a broth culture through a membrane filter of 0.22–0.45 μm.

(The ability to pass through a filter that would normally retain bacteria is a typical characteristic of mycoplasmas.) Dilutions of the filtrate are then plated onto agar to obtain isolated colonies. Each colony should represent the progeny of a single cell that passed through the filter and is therefore a clone. Clones are picked and transferred to broth. The procedure is repeated at least two more times. This technique does not absolutely guarantee the purity of a culture, but the probability is excellent that a triple-cloned culture represents a single mycoplasma culture.

Absence of Cell Wall

Electron microscopy will give clear evidence for the absence of a cell wall, but is not practical for most laboratories. An alternate procedure is to examine a broth culture by phase-contrast or darkfield microscopy to demonstrate pleomorphism. Mycoplasmas will have a variety of sizes and shapes, from small coccoid bodies to large aggregates to fine filaments.

Detection of Bacterial L-Forms

A culture suspected of being a bacterial L-form can be confirmed by five consecutive subcultures in an inhibitor-free broth medium, followed by subculture to an inhibitor-free solid medium to test for reversion from an L-form to a wall-covered bacterial form. Alternatively, colonies on a solid medium can be transferred directly from plate to plate by friction smears. Either technique can be time-consuming for most diagnostic purposes. If a culture has the characteristics of a typical mycoplasma and can be shown both biochemically and serologically to be a known species, this is rather conclusive evidence that the culture is not a bacterial L-form.

Colony Morphology

Most mycoplasma colonies have a "fried egg" morphology on solid media, depending upon the medium and incubation conditions. A dense central core grows down into the medium, and the periphery is primarily surface growth. There are many variations on this theme, ranging from colonies that are all core to those that are nearly all periphery. A few species have no central core. An inoculating loop will easily remove the periphery of a colony, but the central core will remain embedded in the medium. Colonies without cores will be removed entirely.

Mycoplasma colonies can be differentiated from bacterial colonies by a variety of criteria. They are usually smaller (50–500 μm in diameter), have the "fried egg" morphology, and retain the Dienes stain.[30,35] One technique to demonstrate Dienes staining is to excise a 1 cm^2 plug of agar and place it colony-side-up on a glass microscope slide. Gently place a coverslip that has been smeared with Dienes stain on the agar plug. Mycoplasma colonies stain blue and will retain the stain. Most bacterial colonies will remain unstained. The final determination can be made within 30 minutes.

Sterol Requirement

The requirement for sterol separates the non-sterol-dependent acholeplasmas from the sterol-dependent mycoplasmas, ureaplasmas, and spiroplasmas. A direct test for this requirement measures the growth response of the organism to increasing levels of cholesterol.[36,49] An indirect test is based on the measurement of growth inhibition to digitonin.[19] Its results closely parallel those of the direct test, and are easier to obtain. The indirect test is carried out on a solid medium that will support growth of the organism. Flooding the surface of the tilted plate with an appropriately diluted broth culture and removing the excess inoculum will produce a uniform lawn of growth. (The solid medium must contain 10–20% serum, even if the test is done on an organism not requiring sterol for growth.) A digitonin disk is placed on the surface of the medium after it has dried. These disks can be prepared in advance by impregnating 6 mm paper disks with 0.025 ml of a 1.5% (w/v) ethanolic solution of digitonin. They can be used fresh or allowed to dry and then stored at 4°C. Mycoplasmas are sensitive to digitonin and acholeplasmas are resistant. Sensitivity is indicated by a clear zone of inhibition measuring at least 4–5 mm from the edge of the disk to the microbial growth. Resistance is indicated by growth up to the disk or a slight 1–2 mm zone of inhibition.

Biochemical Methods of Identification

The following biochemical tests have proven adequate to characterize most mycoplasma isolates prior to serological identification. The recommendations of the Subcommittee on the Taxonomy of Mycoplasmatales[43] should be consulted for a more complete list of tests.

Glucose Fermentation

Various techniques have been described to determine glucose fermentation in mycoplasmas. These include the determination of glucose disappearance by the glucose oxidase reaction,[15] the determination of acid fermentation products from radioactive glucose, and the determination of hexokinase activity as evidence of the glycolytic pathway.[9] These methods are sensitive and specific, but the simple test based on the determination of a decrease in pH of the growth medium[1] is adequate in most cases. Occasional problems may arise in the interpretation of this test. A slight decrease in pH of uninoculated medium may occur because of the serum or yeast extract components. Non-fermenting mycoplasmas may also cause a slight decrease in pH because of the slight production of acidic products by the metabolism of compounds other than glucose. Suggestions to circumvent these difficulties have included the deletion of yeast extract and the use of 1% (v/v) PPLO serum fraction instead of 10% whole serum. The basal medium should also be pretreated with glucose oxidase and arginine decarboxylase to remove any traces of glucose and arginine.[20] A third problem is that some acholeplasmas will quickly decolorize the phenol red in the medium, hampering detection of a decrease in pH.

Appropriate controls are used to make a valid interpretation of this test. These are an (a) inoculated and (b) an uninoculated test tube of basal medium with the test substrate and (c) an inoculated test tube of basal medium. The inoculum should be 1 ml of a triple-cloned culture actively growing in basal medium. Media can be incubated up to 2 weeks. The pH of the uninoculated basal medium with substrate (b) should have little or no pH shift. A drop of 0.5 pH unit or more in the inoculated basal medium with substrate (a) compared to the inoculated basal medium (c) should be considered a positive reaction. The pH values can be determined by comparison with a set of pH standards ranging from 6.0–8.2. These can be prepared in 0.2 pH unit increments using the basal medium.[1] Each batch of media should have a quality control check with glucose-positive and -negative cultures. If this medium will not support the growth of a particular mycoplasma, a more enriched medium can be substituted. Appropriate inhibitors can be added if desired.

Arginine and Urea Hydrolysis

The procedure for glucose fermentation should be followed with these two modifications: replace glucose with arginine (0.2%) or urea (1%), and adjust the pH of the medium to 7.0. The use of appropriate controls and quality control checks, as for glucose fermentation, will largely overcome problems involved with the interpretation of these tests. A positive test is an alkaline shift of at least a 0.5 pH unit between the two inoculated tubes. Strains that utilize both glucose and arginine sometimes pose a problem with interpretation. The acid produced from the fermentation of compounds other than glucose may mask the alkalinity produced by arginine hydrolysis. The acidic shift initially seen in the basal medium with arginine will often be reversed in time. The pH will then shift into the alkaline range, thereby providing a true result. Other techniques to detect arginine hydrolysis by the determination of the breakdown product citrulline have been described.[5]

Phosphatase Activity

Phosphatase activity is based on the hydrolysis by phosphatase of phenolphthalein diphosphate into free phenolphthalein. Phenolphthalein diphosphate is colorless, whereas phenolphthalein is red in the pH range 9–10. Hydrolysis can be determined using a solid or a liquid medium.[20] Both give comparable results, but the method utilizing a solid medium is less labor intensive.

Petri plates (50 mm diameter) are inoculated in triplicate and incubated at 37°C along with three uninoculated control plates. On days 3, 7, and 14 post-inoculation, one test plate and one control plate are flooded with 5N NaOH. A positive test is indicated by the immediate appearance of red in the medium. A negative test is indicated by little or no color change.

Film and Spot Production

Film and spot production is characteristic of some mycoplasmas, and is produced by colonies growing on a solid medium containing 20% heat-inactivated horse serum. The wrinkled film that develops on the medium surface consists of cholesterol and phospholipids. The tiny black spots that appear beneath and around the colonies are attributed to the deposition of calcium and magnesium salts of fatty acids liberated by the lipolytic activity of mycoplasmas.[18]

Solid[1] medium is inoculated with an actively growing culture and incubated at 37°C. Examination with a dissecting microscope will facilitate early detection. As film and spot production progresses, it can be seen by gross examination. Plates should not be incubated longer than 2 weeks because false positive reactions may occur.

Liquefaction of Inspissated Serum

Proteolytic activity is useful in the characterization of a limited number of mycoplasma species, particularly as a preliminary to final serological identification. Inspissated serum slants are inoculated with an actively growing broth culture. The slants are incubated at 37°C after removal of any excess inoculum. They are examined for 2 weeks for any evidence of liquefaction of the serum-rich slant. Additional tests for proteolytic activity of mycoplasmas involving the hydrolysis of casein[1] and liquefaction of gelatin[17] have been described.

Serological Methods of Identification

Introduction

Two basic groups of serological methods with varying sensitivities and specificities have been used to identify mycoplasmas on a routine diagnostic basis. The first group includes procedures that use living mycoplasmas whose growth or metabolic function can be inhibited by specific antiserum, e.g., growth inhibition and metabolic inhibition tests. The second group involves the identification of mycoplasmas by specific antibody reactions with whole organisms or their antigens, e.g., immunofluorescence. These are the most commonly used methods for species identification. Species that are serologically distinct according to these tests have been shown to share common antigens, which can be demonstrated by double immunodiffusion, growth precipitation, and two-dimensional immunoelectrophoresis. This sharing of antigens occurs among the glycolytic species or among arginine-utilizing species, but only rarely between these two biochemically distinct groups.

The primary problem involved in preparing mycoplasmas as immunogens is the absorption of proteins from the growth medium supplemented with animal serum. The production of antibodies to these media components occurs during immunization. Test antigens that are prepared from other mycoplasma species grown in the same medium will non-specifically cross-react in a number of serological procedures.[27] This is usually not a problem with the growth and metabolic inhibition tests but does occur with immunofluorescence tests.

The most effective way to prevent such non-specific cross-reactivity is to grow the immunogen in a medium containing serum from the animal species to be immunized. This recommendation may be extended to other medium components, e.g., rabbits could be immunized with mycoplasmas grown in rabbit meat infusion broth supplemented with rabbit serum.[47] Not all mycoplasmas grow well in rabbit infusion medium, so an alternate approach is to use a dialysate broth of soy peptone and fresh yeast extract.[26,27] Since not all mycoplasmas can be adapted to grow in rabbit serum, fetal calf serum or bovine serum fraction can be substituted. In addition, other media can be prepared as dialysates. The immunizing and test antigens can also be grown in media with different serum supplements. Acholeplasmas should be grown in serum-free medium.

Organisms are grown to the late log phase in the selected medium and concentrated by centrifugation. After washing three times in buffered saline to remove soluble media components, the organisms are concentrated by resuspending in a small volume of buffered saline. This material can be frozen at −20 to −70°C or used immediately as an immunogen. Inoculation protocols differ[28,39] with the needs of the individual laboratory.

The pre-immunization sera of animals to be immunized should be screened to show that they are not inhibitory to mycoplasmal growth. Rabbit serum often is inhibitory to acholeplasmas.[48] Animals whose sera have precipitation lines in an immunodiffusion test with candidate antigens should not be immunized. Alternatively, the growth inhibition test can be used to evaluate pre-immunization sera.

The growth inhibition test is used to evaluate antisera during immunization trials. Sera that show zones of inhibition of 5 mm or more will usually be satisfactory for other serological tests. The potency of an antiserum that has low or unsatisfactory growth-inhibiting activity can sometimes be increased by concentration.[53] Serum can be frozen at −20°C or lyophilized for long-term storage. Short-term storage at 4°C is adequate if the serum does not evaporate or become contaminated.

Growth Inhibition

The growth inhibition test is based on the observation[14,32] that specific antisera will inhibit the growth of homologous mycoplasmas. Inhibition of growth by specific antisera can occur either on solid or in liquid media. The results of the test on solid media can be observed directly or microscopically. The results in liquid media can be determined indirectly by means of the metabolic inhibition test (see next section).

The growth inhibition test on solid medium has gained widespread acceptance for identification and classification at the species level. It is a species specific test that is economical to perform, rapid to set up, and requires only potent antisera, appropriate growth medium, and a stereo or low-power light microscope. It is probably the best test for identification at the species level, but undiluted or slightly diluted antisera must be used. An antiserum that gives a well-defined zone of inhibition to the homologous strain may inhibit other strains of the same species to a lesser extent. This technique is recommended for the speciation of mycoplasmas but not for the quantitation of antibodies. It is the method of choice for evaluating antisera during immunization trials.

The growth inhibition test is performed on a solid medium using 6 mm filter paper disks impregnated with 0.025 ml antiserum. Reliable results are obtained if a few technical points are observed. High-titered, monospecific antiserum should be used. Preservatives that might inhibit mycoplasma growth should be avoided. Serum can be applied to the disks immediately before use, or the disks can be made up in quantity, dried, and stored at 4°C or −20°C for later use.

The test organism should be a pure culture, i.e., triply cloned through membrane filters. Mixed cultures can lead to erroneous conclusions because a zone of inhibition could be obscured by the growth of an uninhibited organism. The inoculum titer should be in the range of 10^4 to 10^5 colony-forming units (CFU)/ml. Too many organisms will decrease the size of the zone of inhibition whereas too few will give an inconclusive result. A given volume of titered culture can either be spread over the plate with a sterile bent glass rod or allowed to run down the plate (running drop technique). Flooding all or part of a tilted plate and removing the excess inoculum with a Pasteur pipe will always produce a uniform lawn of growth. The surface of the plate should be dry before applying the serum disk. Allow 2 cm^2 of surface area for each disk.

Organisms with rapid growth rates can occasionally yield smaller zones of inhibition. Strategies to overcome this have included incubation at 22–30°C either for the entire length of the test or overnight before transferring the plate to 37°C. Media with suboptimal concentrations of essential components (serum, yeast extract, or bovine serum fraction) will significantly enhance the zone of inhibition. Cutting wells in the agar and filling them with antiserum will also enhance the results.

The zones of inhibition around antiserum disks are not always sharply defined. Breakthrough colonies may be seen within the zone. Judgment is required to determine if the test is valid or should be repeated with a different antiserum. The width of the zone of inhibition, as measured from the edge of the disk to the lawn of mycoplasma growth, should be 5 mm or more. Zones up to 2 mm should be considered equivocal.

In-depth analyses of the technical aspects of this test and its modifications have been presented elsewhere.[11,12,55]

Metabolic Inhibition

The metabolic inhibition test is a growth inhibition technique carried out in liquid medium. It has the specificity of the growth inhibition test using solid medium but is more sensitive. It can be used successfully for the measurement of antibodies to mycoplasmas.

The technique is based upon the fact that mycoplasmas multiplying in a liquid medium containing a specific substrate will metabolize the substrate. The metabolic by-products will alter the pH of the medium as indicated by the change in color of an appropriate pH indicator. The inhibitory activity of homologous antiserum to the mycoplasma under test will decrease the cumulative cell metabolism and therefore indirectly prevent the color change. A microtiter system is used to determine the amount of inhibition of glucose fermentation by glycolytic mycoplasmas,[46] arginine hydrolysis by non-glycolytic mycoplasmas,[33] or urea hydrolysis by ureaplasmas.[34] The titer of a test serum is the highest dilution of serum that prevents a change in color of the medium. This test can be used to identify isolates with known, titered antisera, or to evaluate the potency of a test serum with known cultures.

A variation of the metabolic inhibition test is the tetrazolium reduction inhibition test.[40,41] This test is based on the observation that certain mycoplasmas will reduce colorless 2,3,5-triphenyltetrazolium chloride to its brick-red formazan. This property can be used to demonstrate the metabolic inhibition of mycoplasmas by specific antibody. The test procedure is similar to that of the metabolic inhibition test, but it measures a different metabolic property of the mycoplasma. The inhibition of tetrazolium reduction will result in no color change in the medium. The titer of a test serum is the highest dilution of serum which prevents a color change, i.e., which completely inhibits the reduction of tetrazolium to a red precipitate. This test is useful if an organism is unable to utilize either arginine or glucose, but can reduce tetrazolium. If a mycoplasma is glycolytic and can also reduce tetrazolium, the tetrazolium reduction inhibition titers of antisera are similar to those obtained with the metabolic inhibition test using acid production from glucose as an indicator system. Hence, the two tests are comparable in their sensitivity.

Another variation of the metabolic inhibition test is to combine it with the spiroplasma deformation test. The deformation test[52] is a serological procedure that evaluates the potency of antisera by demonstrating their ability to deform helical spiroplasmas into spheroidal forms. The deformation titer of a test serum is that dilution which completely or partially deforms one-half of the spiroplasmas. The combined test[50,51] is carried out in microtiter plates. The deformation test is read in 30 minutes using darkfield microscopy, and the metabolic inhibition test is read in 3–10 days. Antibody titers observed in these two tests are closely correlated, indicating comparable sensitivity.

The metabolic inhibition test is highly specific and can be used for mycoplasma speciation. Unlike the growth inhibition test, it is highly sensitive. It is more useful for detection of intraspecies antigenic differences than the growth inhibition test since antigenic diversity can be clearly detected.[37] The test is also effective for determining antibody titers using known cultures. It has been used in the classification and characterization of mycoplasmas and in diagnostic and epidemiological studies.

Although the basis for the test is relatively simple, knowledge of the technical aspects is critical for obtaining satisfactory results.[44,54] Results are most reproducible if cultures are divided into aliquots, stored at $-70°C$, and a thawed aliquot is used for each test. Filtering the culture through a 0.45-μm membrane just before freezing to obtain a suspension of single cells is recommended, especially for rapidly growing cultures. Antisera will inhibit the multiplication of individual cells more effectively than that of clumps of organisms. Each thawed aliquot of culture must be titered to determine the appropriate dilution to obtain the 100–1000 color change units (CCU)/unit volume used in the test. The test organism should multiply easily in the test medium and produce an appropriate pH shift or reduction of tetrazolium.

The serum under test and other liquid components of the test must be sterile. Low antibody titers can be obscured by color changes caused by bacterial contaminants in the lower dilutions of serum. Serum from an animal being given antibiotic therapy might inhibit mycoplasma multiplication and mimic the effect of antibody. The strain of a mycoplasma species used in the test may influence the antibody titer since some strains are more capable of detecting antibody than others.[45]

Controls should include a medium control (specific medium minus mycoplasma and test serum), a mycoplasma control (specific medium plus mycoplasma minus test serum), and an endpoint medium control (specific medium with pH adjusted to the desired endpoint, i.e., 0.5 pH units higher or lower than the medium control). The test is read when the medium in the mycoplasma controls is the same color as the endpoint medium controls. Tetrazolium reduction readings are made when mycoplasma controls have a red precipitate. A positive serum of known titer is also run. Results are usually obtained in 1–6 days.

Immunofluorescence

Immunofluorescent staining is an easy and practical technique for the identification of mycoplasmas. Its applications have included the staining of colony impressions on glass slides,[7,10] coverslip preparations from broth cultures,[16] colonies of fastidious mycoplasmas grown on filter membranes,[2,3,4] tissue sections to detect fastidious mycoplasmas,[29,31] and cell cultures to detect mycoplasma infection.[6] One of the most widespread applications is the immunofluorescent staining of colonies on solid media with evaluation by epi-illumination.[13]

Immunofluorescence has been used for the identification of direct agar isolations of mycoplasmas from a variety of sources. It is especially valuable with organisms that are difficult to subculture from the isolation plates. Each mycoplasma colony can be stained to give a representative view of the mycoplasma population of the sample. The purity of cultures can be evaluated, and mixed cultures can be easily detected.

Immunofluorescence is a species specific test like the growth and metabolic inhibition tests and, like metabolic inhibition, is highly sensitive. A microscope equipped with an attachment for incident illumination is required. Identification can be made in a few hours. Cloning of isolates is not a requirement, and the reading of the test is not influenced by inoculum size as long as colonies are not confluent. This is in direct contrast to the growth and metabolic inhibition tests that require quantitated pure cultures and may take days to yield a result.

Both the direct[13] and indirect[38] immunofluorescent staining of colonies on solid media have proven their value for mycoplasma identification. The choice of which technique to use is often dictated by the availability of reagents. The direct test requires a conjugated antiserum specific for each mycoplasma to be tested. The conjugated fluorochrome is usually fluorescein isothiocyanate. Conjugating large numbers of antisera can be time-consuming. The indirect test often requires only one conjugated reagent, an anti-rabbit globulin, since most antisera are produced in rabbits. This conjugate and others directed against the globulins of other species are available commercially. Both tests are specific, but the indirect test is more sensitive and tends to give less non-specific background fluorescence that might interfere with the interpretation of the test. The indirect test also has the potential for screening sera for mycoplasma antibodies.

Working dilutions of antisera and conjugate must be determined before performing the tests. The highest dilution of conjugate giving maximum fluorescence against the homologous strain in a direct test often is not the best working dilution. The homologous fluorescence titer may be one or two dilutions lower since some strains require a higher concentration of antibody than that needed by the strain used in the production of the antiserum. The working dilution of the fluorescein-conjugated anti-rabbit globulin used in the indirect test is determined by box titration[23,24] using a potent positive rabbit antiserum. The plateau endpoint is the highest dilution of conjugate that will give maximum fluorescence against the highest dilution of serum. This plateau endpoint titer is then used to determine the optimal dilution of other antisera.

An entire agar plate need not be stained if the volume of reagents is limited. Excised agar blocks can be transferred to glass slides[38] or microtiter wells[42] for staining. Alternatively, colonies can be stained on the plate after beveled cylinders have been pushed down through the agar. After staining, the cylinders are removed and the agar plugs can be transferred to slides for viewing.

Positive and negative control cultures should be run when unknown isolates are being identified to ensure that the reagents are working properly. Working dilutions of conjugate tend to give diminished fluorescence after multiple freeze/thaw cycles. Plates on which film and spots have developed will give false negative or sub-optimal positive results. Agar plugs exposed only to phosphate buffered saline should be examined for autofluorescence. A control should be included to show that the conjugated anti-rabbit globulin alone does not cause any fluorescence.

Protocols for both tests are standardized,[22] as are the procedures for the fractionation and labeling of antisera.[8,22,25] Detailed discussions of the components of epifluorescent microscopy are also available.[8,25]

References

1. Aluotto BB, Wittler RG, Williams CO, Faber JE: 1970, Standardized bacteriologic techniques for the characterization of Mycoplasma species. Int J Syst Bacteriol 20:35–58.

2. Armstrong CH: 1976, A diagnostically practical approach to isolating and identifying mycoplasmas of porcine origin. Proc Am Assoc Vet Lab Diagn 19:75–91.

3. Armstrong CH: 1977, A diagnostically practical method of isolating and identifying *Mycoplasma hyopneumoniae*. Proc Int Symp Vet Lab Diagn 1:754–771.

4. Armstrong CH, Friis NF: 1981, Isolation of *Mycoplasma flocculare* from swine in the United States. Am J Vet Res 42:1030–1032.

5. Barile MF: 1983, Arginine hydrolysis. In: Methods in Mycoplasmology, Vol. 1. Eds. Razin S, Tully JG, pp. 345–349. Academic Press, New York.

6. Barile MF, Grabowski MW: 1983, Detection and identification of mycoplasmas in infected cell cultures by direct immunofluorescence staining. In: Methods in Mycoplasmology, Vol. 2. Eds. Tully JG, Razin S, pp. 173–181. Academic Press, New York.

7. Carski TR, Shepard CC: 1961, Pleuropneumonia-like (mycoplasma) infections of tissue culture. J Bacteriol 81:626–635.

8. Cherry WB: 1980, Immunofluorescence techniques. In: Manual of Clinical Microbiology, 3rd ed. Ed. Lennette EH, pp. 501–508. Am Soc Microbiol, Washington, D.C.

9. Cirillo VP, Razin S: 1973, Distribution of a phosphoenolpyruvate-dependent sugar phosphotransferase system in mycoplasmas. J Bacteriol 113:212–217.

10. Clark HW, Bailey JS, Fowler RC, Brown T McP: 1963, Identification of Mycoplasmataceae by the fluorescent antibody method. J Bacteriol 85:118.

11. Clyde WA: 1964, Mycoplasma species identification based upon growth inhibition by specific antiserum. J Immunol 92:958–965.

12. Clyde WA: 1983, Growth inhibition tests. In: Methods in Mycoplasmology, Vol. 1. Eds. Razin S, Tully JG, pp. 405–410. Academic Press, New York.

13. Del Giudice RA, Robillard NF, Carski TR: 1967, Immunofluorescence identification of mycoplasma on agar by use of incident illumination. J Bacteriol 93:1205–1209.

14. Edward DG ff., Fitzgerald WA: 1954, Inhibition of growth of pleuropneumoniae-like organisms by antibody. J Pathol Bacteriol 68:23–30.

15. Edward DG ff., Moore WB: 1975, A method for determining the utilization of glucose by mycoplasmas. J Med Microbiol 8:451–454.

16. Ertel PY, Ertel IJ, Somerson NL, Pollack JD: 1970, Immunofluorescence of mycoplasma colonies grown on coverslips. Proc Soc Expt Biol Med 134:441–446.

17. Freundt EA: 1983, Proteolytic activity. In: Methods in Mycoplasmology, Vol. 1. Eds. Razin S, Tully JG, pp. 367–371. Academic Press, New York.

18. Freundt EA: 1983, Film and spot production. In: Methods in Mycoplasmology, Vol. 1. Eds. Razin S, Tully JG, pp. 373–374. Academic Press, New York.

19. Freundt EA, Andrews BE, Erno H, Kunze M, Black FT: 1973, The sensitivity of Mycoplasmatales to sodium-polyanethol-sulfonate and digitonin. Zbl Bakt Hyg, I. Abt Orig A 225:104–112.

20. Freundt EA, Erno H, Lemcke RM: 1979, Identification of mycoplasmas. In: Methods in Microbiology, Vol. 13. Eds. Bergan T, Norris JR, pp. 377–434. Academic Press, New York.

21. Friis NF: 1975, Some recommendations concerning isolation of *Mycoplasma suipneumoniae* and *Mycoplasma flocculare*. Nord Vet Med 27:337–339.

22. Gardella RS, Del Giudice RA, Tully JG: 1983, Immunofluorescence. In: Methods in Mycoplasmology, Vol. 1. Eds. Razin S, Tully JG, pp. 431–439. Academic Press, New York.

23. Hale WL, Bergquist R: 1971, Chessboard analyses with antinuclear antibodies. Ann NY Acad Sci 177:354–360.

24. Hardy PH, Nell EE: 1971, Characteristics of fluorescein-labelled antiglobulin preparations that may affect the fluorescent treponemal antibody absorption test. Am J Clin Pathol 56:181–186.

25. Jones GL, Hebert GA, Cherry WB: 1978, Fluorescent antibody techniques and bacterial applications. HEW Publication (CDC) No. 78-8364.

26. Kenny GE: 1967, Heat-lability and organic solvent-solubility of mycoplasma antigens. Ann NY Acad Sci 143(1):676–681.

27. Kenny GE: 1979, Antigenic determinants. In: The Mycoplasmas, Vol. 1. Eds. Barile MF, Razin S, pp. 351–384. Academic Press, New York.

28. Kenny GE: 1983, Agar precipitin and immunoelectrophoretic methods for detection of mycoplasma antigens. In: Methods in Mycoplasmology, Vol. 1. Eds. Razin S, Tully JG, pp. 441–456. Academic Press, New York.

29. L'Ecuyer C, Boulanger P: 1970, Enzootic pneumonia of pigs: Identification of a causative mycoplasma in infected pigs and in cultures by immunofluorescent staining. Canad J Comp Med 34:38–46.

30. Madoff S: 1960, Isolation and identification of PPLO. Ann NY Acad Sci 79:383–392.

31. Meyling A: 1971, *Mycoplasma suipneumoniae* and *Mycoplasma hyorhinis* demonstrated in pneumonic pig lungs by the fluorescent antibody technique. Acta Vet Scand 12:137–141.

32. Nicol CS, Edward DG ff.: 1953, Role of organisms of the pleuropneumonia group in human genital infections. Br J Vener Dis 29:141–150.

33. Purcell RH, Taylor-Robinson D, Wong DC, Chanock RM: 1966, A color test for the measurement of antibody to the non-acid-forming human mycoplasma species. Am J Epidemiol 84:51–66.

34. Purcell RH, Taylor-Robinson D, Wong DC, Chanock RM: 1966, Color test for the measurement of antibody of T-strain mycoplasmas. J Bacteriol 92:6–12.

35. Razin S: 1983, Identification of mycoplasma colonies. In: Methods in Mycoplasmology, Vol. 1. Eds. Razin S, Tully JG, pp. 373–374. Academic Press, New York.

36. Razin S, Tully JG: 1970, Cholesterol requirement of mycoplasmas. J Bacteriol 102:306–310.

37. Ro LH, Ross RF: 1983, Comparison of *Mycoplasma hyopneumoniae* strains by serologic methods. Am J Vet Res 44:2087–2094.

38. Rosendal S, Black FT: 1972, Direct and indirect immunofluorescence of unfixed and fixed mycoplasma colonies. Acta Path Microbiol Scand, Sect. B 80:615–622.

39. Senterfit LB: 1983, Preparation of antigens and antisera. In: Methods in Mycoplasmology, Vol. 1. Eds. Razin S, Tully JG, pp. 401–404. Academic Press, New York.

40. Senterfit LB: 1983, Tetrazolium reduction inhibition. In: Methods in Mycoplasmology, Vol. 1. Eds. Razin S, Tully JG, pp. 419–421. Academic Press, New York.

41. Senterfit LB, Jensen KE: 1966, Antimetabolic antibodies to *Mycoplasma pneumoniae* measured by tetrazolium reduction inhibition. Proc Soc Exp Biol Med 122:786–790.

42. Stemke GW, Robertson JA: 1981, Modified colony indirect epifluorescence test for serotyping *Ureaplasma urealyticum* and an adaption to detect common antigenic specificity. J Clin Microbiol 14:582–584.

43. Subcommittee on the Taxonomy of Mollicutes (1979). Proposal of minimal standards

for description of new species of the class Mollicutes. Int J Syst Bacteriol 29:172–180.

44. Taylor-Robinson D: 1983, Metabolism inhibition tests. In: Methods in Mycoplasmology, Vol. 1. Eds. Razin S, Tully JG, pp. 411–417. Academic Press, New York.

45. Taylor-Robinson D, Berry DM: 1969, The evaluation of the metabolic inhibition technique for the study of *Mycoplasma gallisepticum*. J Gen Microbiol 55:127–137.

46. Taylor-Robinson D, Purcell RH, Wong DC, Chanock RM: 1966, A color test for the measurement of antibody to certain mycoplasma species based on the inhibition of acid production. J Hyg 64:91–104.

47. Taylor-Robinson D, Somerson NL, Turner HC, Chanock RM: 1963, Serological relationships among human mycoplasmas as shown by complement fixation and gel diffusion. J Bacteriol 85:1261–1273.

48. Tully JG: 1979, Special features of the acholeplasmas. In: The Mycoplasmas, Vol. 1. Eds. Barile MF, Razin S, pp. 431–449. Academic Press, New York.

49. Tully JG: 1983, Tests for digitonin sensitivity and sterol requirement. In: Methods in Mycoplasmology, Vol. 1. Eds. Razin S, Tully JG, pp. 355–362. Academic Press, New York.

50. Williamson DL: 1983, The combined deformation-metabolism inhibition test. In: Methods in Mycoplasmology, Vol. 1. Eds. Razin S, Tully JG, pp. 477–483. Academic Press, New York.

51. Williamson DL, Tully JG, Whitcomb RF: 1979, Serological relationships of spiroplasmas as shown by combined deformation and metabolic inhibition tests. Int J Syst Bacteriol 29:345–351.

52. Williamson DL, Whitcomb RF, Tully JG: 1978, The spiroplasma deformation test, a new serological method. Curr Microbiol 1:203–207.

53. Windsor GD, Trigwell JA: 1976, Method for concentrating antisera for preparing mycoplasma growth inhibition discs. Res Vet Sci 20:221–222.

54. World Health Organization (1975). "The Metabolism-Inhibition Test," Working Doc VPH/MIC/75.6. Working Group of the FAO/WHO Programme on Comparative Mycoplasmology, WHO, Geneva.

55. World Health Organization (1976). "The Growth Inhibition Test," Working Doc VPH/MIC/76.7. Working Group of the FAO/WHO Programme on Comparative Mycoplasmology, WHO, Geneva.

Appendix A3.1

Basal Medium

Heart infusion broth (Difco)	84.50 ml
Horse serum, heat-inactivated (56°C for 30 minutes)	5.00 ml
Swine serum, acid-adjusted, heat-inactivated (56°C for 30 minutes)	5.00 ml
Yeast extract, fresh	5.00 ml
Phenol red, 1% (w/v)	0.50 ml

Adjust to pH 7.6 for glucose fermentation and pH 7.0 for arginine and urea hydrolysis. Sterilize by filtration and dispense 5 ml per screw-capped test tube.

Test Substrate (per 100 ml basal medium)

Glucose	1.0 gm
Arginine	0.2 gm
Urea	1.0 gm

Yeast Extract, fresh[21]

Fleischmann's dry yeast, type 2040	125 gm
Water, deionized, distilled	750 ml

Mix and place in 37°C water bath for 20 minutes. Heat immediately to 95°C for 5 minutes. After cooling, centrifuge at 1000 × g for 30 minutes. Dispense the supernatant fluid in convenient aliquots and autoclave at 115°C for 5 minutes. Store at −20°C for up to 3 months.

Acid-adjusted Swine Serum

1. Adjust the pH of the swine serum with lN HCl to 4.3–4.5. Do not go below 4.2.
2. Allow serum to stand 1 to 18 hours at 4°C.
3. Centrifuge at 2000 rpm for 30 minutes. Discard sediment.
4. Centrifuge at a higher speed if necessary to remove any additional suspended material.
5. Adjust pH to 7.0 with lN NaOH.
6. Store at −20°C.

Glucose Oxidase – Arginine Decarboxylase Treatment

1. Add 25 mg glucose oxidase (Type II, Sigma) to 1000 ml heart infusion broth.
2. Adjust pH to 5.4–5.6 with concentrated HCl.
3. Aerate for 1 hour at 35–38°C with compressed air or oxygen.
4. Add 25 mg arginine decarboxylase (Sigma).
5. Aerate as in step 3.
6. Cool broth to room temperature.
7. Adjust to desired pH, 7.0 or 7.6.
8. Autoclave for 20 minutes to destroy the activity of added enzymes.

Phosphatase Medium

Heart infusion agar (Difco)	74 ml

Horse serum, sterile, heat-inactivated (60°C for 1 hour)	20 ml
Yeast extract solution (sterile, heat-inactivated 60°C for 1 hour)	5 ml
Phenolphthalein diphosphate, 1%, (w/v)	1 ml

Adjust pH to 7.8 before autoclaving heart infusion agar. Cool to 56°C and aseptically add other ingredients. Pour 8–10 ml per 15 × 60 mm petri plate.

Film and Spot Medium

Heart infusion agar (Difco)	75 ml
Horse serum, sterile, heat-inactivated, (56°C for 30 minutes)	20 ml
Yeast extract solution, sterile	5 ml

Adjust pH to 7.8 before autoclaving heart infusion agar. Cool to 56°C and add other ingredients. Pour 8–10 ml per 15 × 60 mm petri plate.

Inspissated Serum

Heart infusion broth (Difco)	16.0 ml
Horse serum, sterile	60.0 ml
Yeast extract solution, sterile	1.6 ml
Water, sterile	2.4 ml

Adjust pH to 7.8 before autoclaving heart infusion broth. Cool to 56°C and add other ingredients. Dispense the medium in 3 ml volumes into sterile 13 × 100 mm screw-capped tubes. Loosen the caps, place tubes in a slanted position, and inspissate for 45 minutes at 80°C.

CHAPTER 4

Avian Mycoplasmas

S. H. KLEVEN

Numerous species of avian mycoplasma have been described. Table 4.1, adapted from Jordan[16] with data from other sources,[7,8,10,12] lists these species along with their biochemical reactions and usual host. Three are commonly recognized as poultry pathogens: *Mycoplasma gallisepticum, M. synoviae,* and *M. meleagridis. M. gallisepticum* is a cause of respiratory disease and decreased egg production in chickens, turkeys, and other avian species, and it is the most economically important of the avian mycoplasmas.[32] Severe airsacculitis, coughing, rales, and poor growth may be observed in broilers or turkeys, with heavy condemnations from airsacculitis at processing. Swollen sinuses are commonly seen in turkeys. *M. synoviae* causes lesions of synovitis in chickens, turkeys, and other species, and may also be involved in respiratory disease.[22] *M. meleagridis,* found only in turkeys, causes respiratory disease in young turkeys, and is involved in stunting, poor feathering, and leg problems.[30] All three of the pathogenic avian mycoplasmas are egg-transmitted, and may be spread laterally by direct or indirect contact. The mode of egg transmission of *M. meleagridis* is venereal; infection of the male phallus results in contaminated semen, which contaminates the oviduct of the female.

M. gallisepticum, M. synoviae, and *M. meleagridis* are covered by control programs administered under the auspices of the National Poultry Improvement Plan.[2] Breeder replacements are tested and certified as clean after negative serological tests. All major breeds of commercial chickens and turkeys in the United States are essentially free of infection. Outbreaks of *M. gallisepticum* and *M. synoviae* in breeding stocks, broiler-type chickens, and in commercial turkeys are sporadic but are relatively infrequent. When grandparent breeder flocks or genetic lines become infected, the

31

Table 4.1.   Characteristics of avian mycoplasmas

Mycoplasma Species	Usual Host	Glucose Fermentation	Arginine Hydrolysis	Phosphatase Activity
A. laidlawii	Various	+	−	+ or −
M. anatis	Duck	+	−	+
M. anseris	Goose	−	+	−
M. cloacale	Turkey	−	+	−
M. columbinasale	Pigeon	−	+	+
M. columbinum	Pigeon	−	+	−
M. columborale	Pigeon	+	−	−
M. gallinarum	Chicken	−	+	−
M. gallinaceum	Chicken	+	−	−
M. gallisepticum	Chicken and turkey	+	−	−
M. gallopavonis	Turkey	+	−	−
M. glycophilum	Chicken	+	−	+ or −
M. iners	Chicken	−	+	−
M. iowae	Turkey	+	+	−
M. lipofaciens	Chicken	+	+	−
M. meleagridis	Turkey	−	+	+
M. pullorum	Chicken	+	−	−
M. synoviae	Chicken and turkey	+	−	−

flock is slaughtered. Multiplier breeder flocks may be slaughtered, but are kept for breeding purposes under some situations. With the advent of multi-age commercial egg production sites, *M. synoviae* and *M. gallisepticum* infection have become relatively common in commercial layer chickens. Egg production losses due to *M. gallisepticum* infection in commercial layers may be controlled by vaccination, either with an inactivated, oil-emulsion bacterin or live vaccine; *M. synoviae* infection in layers is usually considered to be economically insignificant. A relatively high percentage of commercial turkeys are infected with *M. meleagridis,* with variable economic effects. With all of the pathogenic avian mycoplasmas, the severity of the clinical syndrome may depend on the virulence of the mycoplasma strain involved, the age and type of bird, stress, management, weather, and concurrent infections (such as Newcastle disease, infectious bronchitis, and *E. coli*).

Two other avian mycoplasma species have been reported as pathogenic under some conditions. Some strains of *M. gallinarum* have been involved in respiratory disease with airsacculitis in young chickens, both by challenge and under field conditions.[20] *M. iowae* causes embryo mortality in turkeys, both experimentally and under natural conditions; and stunting, poor feathering, leg problems, and tenosynovitis have been produced experimentally.[9] *M. iowae* is egg-transmitted in turkeys.

4. Avian Mycoplasmas *Kleven* **33**

Serology

Screening of poultry flocks for infection with the pathogenic myco-plasmas is generally accomplished with the serum plate agglutination (SPA) test.[2] Generally, 10% of the flock or a minimum of 300 birds are tested before the onset of egg production, and approximately 30 birds per flock are tested every 60–90 days thereafter.

The SPA test is quick, inexpensive, and highly sensitive. Infected birds may test positive as early as 7–10 days after infection. The test involves the use of specific stained antigens for *M. gallisepticum, M. synoviae,* and *M. meleagridis,* respectively. Antigens are available commercially (Solvay Animal Health, Inc., Charles City, IA; and Intervet America, Millsboro, DE). Approximately 0.02 ml of serum and 0.03 ml of antigen are mixed on a glass plate. The plate is rotated for 2–3 minutes, and the tests are exam-ined for visible clumping.[23] Antigens obtained from various sources may differ in sensitivity and specificity,[5] and there are also batch-to-batch varia-tions.

The greatest disadvantage of the SPA test is low specificity (false posi-tive reactions). These have been related to medium components, primarily serum, adhering to the surface of the mycoplasma organisms used to pre-pare the antigen, although false positive reactions may often be unex-plained.[5] False positive reactions are commonly seen after chickens or tur-keys have been vaccinated with inactivated oil emulsion vaccines against other infectious agents, especially if there are remnants of serum in the vaccine.[15] Such false positive reactions may persist up to 4–8 weeks or longer after vaccination. Production of agglutination antigens in medium substituting artificial liposomes for serum may result in agglutination anti-gens of improved specificity.[1] In addition to false positive reactions related to medium components, cross-reacting antigens may be shared between mycoplasma species or between mycoplasmas and bacteria. Several cross-reacting antigens between *M. gallisepticum* and *M. synoviae* have been found using immunoblotting analysis. Also, birds inoculated with *Staphy-lococcus aureus* reacted with several antigens of *M. gallisepticum* on im-munoblots.[4] The SPA test for *M. synoviae* in turkeys is insensitive in some cases, and infected flocks may be missed without further testing. Flocks with SPA reactors should be confirmed as positive or negative with the hemagglutination inhibition (HAI) test, serum plate agglutination or other acceptable serological test, or by culture. Some laboratories prefer to use serum dilutions with the SPA for confirming reactors. Serial two-fold dilu-tions of the serum are made in a buffer such as phosphate buffered saline, and the SPA test is conducted on the diluted sera. Sera that react at 1:8 or 1:10 or greater are considered positive. Overall, the SPA dilution system works well, but it should be remembered that weak but specific SPA reactors may be negative with the serum dilution test, and strong false positive reactors may react at 1:8 or greater.

Agglutination reactors are generally confirmed with the HAI test. Tests are usually conducted in microtiter plates, using 4 hemagglutinating units of antigen per test.[2,23] Generally, HAI titers of 1:40 to 1:80 or greater are considered positive, but results must be interpreted on a flock basis. The HAI test is considered to be highly specific, but less sensitive than the SPA test. Infected birds may not test positive until 3 weeks or longer after infection. In addition, there is antigenic variation among *M. gallisepticum* strains as measured by HAI. Antigen prepared from one *M. gallisepticum* strain may not detect HAI antibodies in chickens infected with a different strain.[21]

ELISA test systems have also been developed in several laboratories,[3,25,29] and commercial test kits are available (IDEXX, Portland, ME; Kirkegaard and Perry Laboratories, Gaithersburg, MD). Such systems are reliable in detecting antibodies against *M. gallisepticum* or *M. synoviae*. They detect antibodies at about the same time after infection as the HAI test. Unfortunately, they also tend to give false positive reactions, but these problems are rapidly being eliminated by the use of improved antigen preparations or other procedures.

In many situations, serological testing may not give a definitive diagnosis, especially when positive agglutination reactions cannot be confirmed by HAI testing. In such cases retesting may be required. In that situation, isolation and identification of the organism may lead to a faster and more definitive diagnosis than repeated serological testing.

No serological test systems are available for avian mycoplasmas other than *M. gallisepticum, M. synoviae,* and *M. meleagridis.*

Isolation

Since the pathogenic avian mycoplasmas persist for long periods in the upper respiratory tract, tracheas or palatine clefts are preferred sites for culture, although tissues showing lesions (air sacs, sinuses, joints, etc.) should be cultured as well. In many cases the organisms are cleared from lesions after a few weeks, but may persist in the upper respiratory tract. In the case of *M. meleagridis,* it may be useful to culture the vagina or phallus of breeding-age turkeys, and the cloaca may be a useful site for isolating *M. iowae. M. iowae* may also be readily isolated from the tissues of dead embryos.

A modification of Frey's medium[13] supports the growth of all recognized avian mycoplasmas, and is the preferred medium. A formulation is given in Table 4.2. However, a medium based on PPLO broth (Difco)[23] may be more efficient for the primary isolation of *M. meleagridis* and *M. iowae.*

Table 4.2.   Frey's medium for the isolation of avian mycoplasmas

Mycoplasma broth base[a]	22.5 g
Dextrose	3.0 g
Swine serum	120.0 ml
Cysteine hydrochloride[b]	0.1 g
Nicotinamide adenine dinucleotide (NAD)[b]	0.1 g
Phenol red (1%)	2.5 ml
Thallium acetate (10%)[c]	5.0 ml
Penicillin G potassium[d]	1,000,000 units
Distilled water	QS 1000.0 ml

Adjust pH to 7.8 with 20% NaOH, and filter-sterilize.

Note: For agar medium use 1% of a purified agar such as ionagar #2, Noble agar, or Difco purified agar. All components except cysteine/NAD, serum, and penicillin are sterilized by autoclaving at 121°C for 15 min. Cool to 50°C and aseptically add the above components, which have been presterilized by filtration and warmed to 50°C. Mix and pour plates to a depth of approximately 5 mm.
   [a]Gibco Diagnostics, Madison, Wisconsin.
   [b]Reduced NAD is required for *M. synoviae* only. A 1% solution of each is mixed in equal parts, and 20 ml is added per liter of medium.
   [c]For potentially contaminated specimens, add an extra 20 ml of 1% thallium acetate per liter of medium to bring total concentration to 1:1500.
   [d]For potentially contaminated material, an extra 2 million units may be added per liter of medium. 1 g of ampicillin per liter of medium will substitute.

Cotton swabs from trachea, air sac, or other tissue (or approximately 0.1 ml of fluid from swollen sinuses or joints) are inoculated into 3–5 ml of broth medium, and the swab is discarded. For *M. meleagridis* and *M. iowae,* direct inoculation on agar plates may be more effective than inoculation of broth. Incubation is at 37°C. Ordinarily, aerobic incubation is sufficient, although some laboratories may prefer to use a candle jar. For *M. synoviae, M. gallisepticum,* and other glucose fermenters, cultures are incubated until the phenol red indicator changes to orange or yellow and then plates are inoculated. For non-fermenters, cultures are plated at about 5 days of incubation and again at about 10–14 days. Agar plates can be divided into sections so that 6–8 cultures can be inoculated on a single agar plate. Cotton swabs or Pasteur pipets can be used. Plates are incubated in a closed jar to prevent dehydration.

Agar plates are examined for mycoplasma colonies under low power magnification (about 35×) with an ordinary light microscope with the light intensity reduced, or with a dissecting microscope. With several of the non-pathogenic species, such as *Acholeplasma, M. gallinarum,* or *M. gallinaceum,* colonies may be observed as early as 24 hours postinoculation; with the pathogenic species, *M. gallisepticum, M. synoviae,* and *M. meleagridis,* colonies are usually present after 4–5 days of incubation at

37°C, but in some instances they may be present after 3 days. Mixed cultures are common, especially in multi-age commercial layers. The most commonly encountered non-pathogenic species are *M. gallinarum* and *M. gallinaceum.* Hyperimmune serum against *M. gallinarum* and *M. gallinaceum* may be added to the broth medium to isolate the slower-growing pathogenic mycoplasma species.

Although biochemical reactions may be useful at times, isolates are ordinarily identified by serological methods, using hyperimmune serum prepared in rabbits.[28] The most commonly used procedures are growth inhibition,[11] immunodiffusion,[24] and immunofluorescence,[6,14] as detailed in Chapter 3.

Differentiation of Strains

M. gallisepticum strains differ in virulence[31] and antigenicity.[21] Additional strain variation has been detected by polyacrylamide gel electrophoresis of mycoplasmal proteins,[18] by restriction endonuclease analysis of DNA,[19,27] and by Southern blot hybridization using a DNA probe prepared from the ribosomal RNA gene of *M. capricolum.*[33] DNA probes have been constructed that are both strain specific and species specific,[17,26] and may be useful in the future for rapid detection of mycoplasmal DNA in clinical specimens.

Such techniques may be useful for differentiation of strains for epidemiological studies. It is likely that similar strain variations will be shown for *M. synoviae, M. meleagridis,* and perhaps the other avian mycoplasmas.

References

1. Ahmad I, Kleven SH, Avakian AP, Glisson JR: 1988, Sensitivity and specificity of *Mycoplasma gallisepticum* agglutination antigens prepared from medium with artificial liposomes substituting for serum. Avian Dis 32:519–526.

2. Anon: 1985, National poultry improvement plan and auxiliary provisions. Publication APHIS 91–40. Animal and Plant Health Inspection Service, US Dept of Agriculture, Hyattsville, MD.

3. Ansari AA, Taylor RF, Chang TS: 1983, Application of enzyme-linked immunosorbent assay for detecting antibody to *Mycoplasma gallisepticum* infections in poultry. Avian Dis 27:21–35.

4. Avakian AP, Kleven SH: 1990, The humoral immune response of chickens to *Mycoplasma gallisepticum* and *Mycoplasma synoviae* studied by immunoblotting. Vet Microbiol 24:155–169.

5. Avakian AP, Kleven SH, Glisson JR: 1988, Evaluation of the specificity and sensitivity of two commercial ELISA kits, the serum plate agglutination test, and hemagglutination

inhibition test for antibodies formed in response to *Mycoplasma gallisepticum.* Avian Dis 32:262–272.

6. Baas EJ, Jasper DE: 1972, Agar block technique for identification of mycoplasma by use of fluorescent antibody. Applied Microbiol 23:1097–1100.

7. Bradbury JM, Forrest M: 1984, *Mycoplasma cloacale,* a new species isolated from a turkey. Int J Syst Bacteriol 34:389–392.

8. Bradbury JM, Forrest M, Williams A: 1983. *Mycoplasma lipofaciens,* a new species of avian origin. Int J Syst Bacteriol 33:329–335.

9. Bradbury JM, Ideris A, Tin Tun Oo: 1988, *Mycoplasma iowae* infection in young turkeys. Avian Path 17:149–171.

10. Bradbury JM, Jordan FTW, Shimizu T, Stipkovits L, Varga Z: 1988, *Mycoplasma anseris* sp. nov. found in geese. Int J Syst Bacteriol 38:74–76.

11. Clyde WA, Jr: 1983, Growth inhibition tests. In: Methods in Mycoplasmology, Vol. 1, Mycoplasma Characterization. Eds. Razin S, Tully JG, pp. 405–410. Academic Press, New York, NY.

12. Forrest M, Bradbury JM: 1984, *Mycoplasma glycophilum,* a new species of avian origin. J Gen Microbiol 130:597–603.

13. Frey ML, Hanson RP, Anderson, DP: 1968, A medium for the isolation of avian mycoplasmas. Amer J Vet Res 29:2163–2171.

14. Gardella RS, DelGiudice RA, Tully JG: 1983, Immunofluorescence. In: Methods in Mycoplasmology, Vol. 1, Mycoplasma characterization. Eds. Razin S, Tully JG, pp. 431–439. Academic Press, New York, NY.

15. Glisson JR, Dawe JF, Kleven SH: 1984, The effect of oil-emulsion vaccines on the occurrence of nonspecific plate agglutination reactions for *Mycoplasma gallisepticum* and *M. synoviae.* Avian Dis 28:397–405.

16. Jordan FTW: 1983, Recovery and Identification of Avian Mycoplasmas. In: Methods in Mycoplasmology, Vol. 2, Diagnostic Mycoplasmology. Eds. Tully JG, Razin S, pp. 69–79. Academic Press, New York, NY.

17. Khan MI, Kirkpatrick BC, Yamamoto R: 1987, A *Mycoplasma gallisepticum* strain-specific DNA probe. Avian Dis 31:907–909.

18. Khan MI, Lam KM, Yamamoto R: 1987, *Mycoplasma gallisepticum* strain variations detected by sodium dodecyl sulfate-polyacrylamide gel electrophoresis. Avian Dis 31:315–320.

19. Kleven SH, Browning GF, Bulach DM, Ghiocas E, Morrow CJ, Whithear KG: 1988, Examination of *Mycoplasma gallisepticum* strains using restriction endonuclease DNA analysis and DNA-DNA hybridization. Avian Path 17:559–570.

20. Kleven SH, Eidson CS, Fletcher OJ: 1987, Airsacculitis induced in broilers with a combination of *Mycoplasma gallinarum* and respiratory viruses. Avian Dis 22:707–716.

21. Kleven SH, Morrow CJ, Whithear KG: 1988, Comparison of *Mycoplasma gallisepticum* strains by hemagglutination inhibition and restriction endonuclease analysis. Avian Dis 32:731–741.

22. Kleven SH, Rowland GN, Olson NO: 1991, Avian mycoplasmosis. *Mycoplasma synoviae* infection. In: Diseases of Poultry, 9th ed. Eds. Calnek BW, Barnes HI, Beard CW, Reid WM, Yoder HW Jr, pp. 223–231. Iowa State University Press, Ames, IA.

23. Kleven SH, Yoder HW, Jr: 1989, Mycoplasmosis. In: A Laboratory Manual for the Isolation and Identification of Avian Pathogens, 3rd ed. Eds. Purchase HG, Arp LH, Domermuth CH, Pearson JE, pp. 57–62. American Association of Avian Pathologists, Kennett Square, PA.

24. Nonomura I, Yoder HW, Jr: 1977, Identification of avian mycoplasma isolates by the agar-gel precipitin test. Avian Dis 21:370–381.

25. Opitz HM, Duplessis JB, Cyr MJ: 1983, Indirect micro-enzyme-linked immunosorbent assay for the detection of antibodies to *Mycoplasma synoviae* and *M. gallisepticum.* Avian Dis 27:773–786.

26. Santha M, Burg K, Rasko I, Stipkovits L: 1987, A species-specific DNA probe for the detection of *Mycoplasma gallisepticum*. Infection and Immunity 55:2857–2859.

27. Santha M, Lukacs K, Burg K, Stipkovits L: 1988, Intraspecies genotypic heterogeneity among *Mycoplasma gallisepticum* strains. Appl Env Microbiol 54:607–609.

28. Senterfit LB: 1983, Preparation of antigens and antisera. In: Methods in Mycoplasmology, Vol. 1, Mycoplasma Characterization. Eds. Razin S and Tully JG, pp. 401–404. Academic Press, New York, NY.

29. Talkington FD, Kleven SH, Brown J: 1985, An enzyme-linked immunosorbent assay for the detection of antibodies to *Mycoplasma gallisepticum* in experimentally infected chickens. Avian Dis 29:53–70.

30. Yamamoto R: 1991, Avian mycoplasmosis. *Mycoplasma meleagridis* infection. In: Diseases of Poultry, 9th ed. Eds. Calnek BW, Barnes HJ, Beard CW, Reid WM, Yoder HW Jr, pp. 212–223. Iowa State University Press, Ames, IA.

31. Yoder HW, Jr: 1986, A historical account of the diagnosis and characterization of strains of *Mycoplasma gallisepticum* of low virulence. Avian Dis 30:510–518.

32. Yoder HW, Jr: 1991, Avian mycoplasmosis. *Mycoplasma gallisepticum* infection. In: Diseases of Poultry, 9th ed. Eds. Calnek BW, Barnes HJ, Beard CW, Reid WM, Yoder HW Jr, pp. 198–212. Iowa State University Press, Ames, IA.

33. Yogev D, Levisohn S, Kleven SH, Halachmi D, Razin S: 1988, Ribosomal RNA gene probes to detect intraspecies heterogeneity in *Mycoplasma gallisepticum* and *M. synoviae*. Avian Dis 32:220–231.

CHAPTER 5

Bovine Mycoplasmas

Contagious Bovine Pleuropneumonia

S. P. SAHU
R. J. YEDLOUTSCHNIG

C ontagious bovine pleuropneumonia (CBPP) is a highly infectious acute or chronic disease primarily affecting cattle and domesticated water buffalo under natural conditions. It is characterized by edema of interlobular and alveolar tissues of the lung as well as a sero-fibrinous pleuritis, and is caused by a pleomorphic filterable organism classified as *Mycoplasma mycoides* subsp. *mycoides* (*M. mycoides*).

The disease was first reported from Germany in 1693. It spread rapidly over the whole of Europe and from there was conveyed to South Africa, Australia, the Far East, and the United States via infected cattle. Eradication of CBPP has been achieved during the past century in Europe, North America, South Africa, and Australia, but it remains a serious problem in some territories of Africa south of the Sahara, in limited areas of Asia, and recently in parts of China and Mongolia.[22]

The disease usually spreads among susceptible animals by inhalation of aerosols. New outbreaks may result when infected particles are released by respiratory expulsion from pulmonary sequestra of "carrier animals." The incubation period in the acute stage is usually 3–6 weeks, but may be as long as 3 months or longer under natural conditions.[35]

The causative agent of CBPP belongs to the order Mycoplasmatales, class Mollicutes formerly *Asterococcus mycoides,* now *M. mycoides.* Mycoplasmas are small pleomorphic organisms that have been cultivated in a suitable, cell-free medium. Ultrafiltration studies indicate these organisms are 125–175 nm in diameter, which is comparable to many filterable viruses. They do not possess a true cell wall, are penicillin resistant, and grow readily outside cell systems in serum-enriched media or on agar plates.[32]

Clinical Signs

Many cases of CBPP are subclinical and cannot be detected. Signs which do develop are normally attributed to lesions that develop in the thoracic cavity. The acute form progresses rapidly, with a sudden febrile response of 40.5°C or more, anorexia, agalactia, and evidence of severe thoracic pain. Coughing may be noticed only following exercise. Breathing may be shallow and rapid, auscultation may reveal gurgling sounds and pleuritic friction to areas of dullness when large portions of the lung are involved. In the most severe stages, the affected animal stands with neck extended and back arched, with the mouth open gasping for breath.

Subacute and chronic forms are also common. The clinical signs may only be dullness, intermittent fever, and a mild cough. The chronic cases often develop into latent carriers when the lung lesions wall off and form sequestra. These carriers are often the cause of continuing spread of the disease. Suspected cases can usually be confirmed only by laboratory test. Young and old animals are most often affected. The young are more prone to develop arthritic lesions rather than pneumonic lesions. The incubation period is highly variable; variation from 20–120 days is documented. The disease normally spreads slowly and insidiously.

Pathogenesis

The primary site of CBPP infection is the thoracic cavity, and infection is solely by aerosol exposure. Experimental infection can be effected by endobronchial intubation of viable broth cultures of *M. mycoides,* aerosol spray, intranasal instillation, or direct contact with actively infected cattle.[1,8,37]

M. mycoides produces natural infections in cattle and water buffalo (*Bubalu bubalus*), but not the wild buffalo (*Syncerus caffer*).[35] Wild bovid species are susceptible (experimentally), but are not known to spread CBPP in nature. Horses, donkeys, and pigs are resistant to *M. mycoides.* Mice are susceptible by experimental inoculation.[19,38]

Strains of *M. mycoides* of the "large colony" type have been isolated from goats and are serologically indistinguishable from the "small colony" *M. mycoides* that produces CBPP in cattle. There is no evidence that the "large colony" *M. mycoides* affects cattle nor that CBPP spreads from goats to cattle. Another mycoplasma, *M. mycoides* subsp. *capri,* produces contagious caprine pleuropneumonia but is non-infective for cattle.

Postmortem Lesions

Signs of natural disease are usually restricted to the respiratory system. The pleural cavity of acutely infected animals may contain 10–20 liters of fluid. The visceral pleura is infected and covered with large deposits of fibrin. Fluid that distends the intralobular spaces and subpleural tissues runs out of incised infected lobes and rapidly coagulates upon exposure to air. Progressive pneumonia develops, which results in death in acute cases. Early pneumonic lesions are characterized by solidification of part of a lobe, a whole lobe, or even more than one lobe of one lung. In the usual acute cases only one lung is involved. Though pulmonary lesions may be bilateral, they are never symmetrical as seen with East coast fever and pasteurellosis.

Lung lesions in acute CBPP are caused by fluid distending the intralobular spaces, giving the lobe a characteristic marbled appearance. The septa often appear beaded due to presence of distended lymph spaces. Necrotic areas that develop during the acute phase tend to become encapsulated by a thick layer of fibrin that forms characteristic sequestra, which may persist for a long time. A lesion may also be absorbed or become a liquified abscess.[2,16,23]

Adhesions between the lung and thoracic wall may become so extensive that the lung must be dissected out. In relatively resistant animals, only a small area of a lung lobe may be affected. In these cases, the lesions may be more easily palpated than seen. Lymph nodes in the thoracic cavity often become enlarged and appear moist when incised.

Location of the affected lung lobe may assist in a differential diagnosis. Any portion(s) of the lung may be affected, and cutting through the palpable mass usually reveals the characteristic "marbled" appearance associated with CBPP lesions.

Diagnosis

Clinical diagnosis may be very difficult unless CBPP is suspected in an endemic area where symptoms associated with pleuropneumonia exist, or suspected cases were observed in an abattoir. In general, cattle, zebu, bison, yak, and domestic buffaloes are affected, whereas CBPP has not been confirmed in the camel, giraffe, wild buffalo, or large antelopes.[35]

Postmortem diagnosis is aided by the "marbled" appearance of lung lesions due to distension of the interlobular septa and hepatization, along with exudative pleurisy. In chronic cases, sequestra may be observed or palpated, and may be mistaken as tuberculosis or some other chronic bacterial disease. The most important procedure at necropsy is to examine the entire lung by palpation, as some lesions may be as small as 1 or 2 cm. Suspicious cases must be confirmed by laboratory studies and differentiated from pasteurellosis, tuberculosis, East coast fever or any other condition affecting the thoracic cavity and/or organs.

All samples should be transported on wet ice or ice gel packs. Samples may be transported with or without media, but always insure that when media is utilized, *no inhibitors* are used. Appropriate samples from live animal include nasal swabs, nasal discharge, thoracic fluid (collected by paracentesis between the 7th and 8th rib), and 10 ml of whole blood. Appropriate samples from dead animals include lung lesion, thoracic fluid, draining lymph nodes, and bronchial lesions. A lung lesion should be submitted in 10% formalin.

Isolation

Direct isolation on agar plates may be done by spreading a few drops of lung "lymph," pleural fluid, or lung homogenate onto the agar surface. Also, a direct smear from the cut surface of a lymph node or lung can be made. The plates should be incubated at 37°C in a humid incubator. A 10% suspension of each tissue should be prepared in sterile broth media, and five 10-fold serial dilutions made in brain-heart infusion broth. A 0.1 ml amount from each tube is streaked onto agar plates, which are incubated at 37°C. Similar titrations should be made and cultured from liquid samples.

Broth cultures will appear milky or cloudy in 3–7 days and should be streaked onto agar plates for positive identification of mycoplasma colonies. Colonies on agar have a typical "fried egg" appearance and vary from 10μ to 600μ in diameter. They are so transparent that they are easily overlooked, and are best observed by checking daily for 5–7 days using a low-power microscope.

M. mycoides is considered relatively easy to isolate and cultivate in suitable media supplemented with proper sera, in comparison with some other mycoplasma species. Broth cultures may require approximately 7 days to obtain optimum growth, and may need subinoculation to fresh media.

If confirmation requires staining, a block of agar supporting colonies is placed face down on a microscope slide, which is then carefully immersed in Bouin's fluid. After 15 minutes the colonies have become attached to the slide. The agar block is removed and the slide washed thoroughly with distilled water buffered to pH 7. Then one of two methods is used:

1. May-Grünwald-Giemsa stain — Stain the slide by the standard procedure and examine at 16–40× or 100× if fine detail is necessary.
2. Dienes' staining — Composition of the stain:

methylene blue	2.50 g
azur II	1.25 g
maltose	10.00 g
sodium carbonate	0.25 g
benzoic acid	0.20 g
distilled water, QS to 100 ml.	

a) The stain is spread on coverslips measuring 22 × 22 mm, which are then allowed to dry.
b) Blocks of agar (bearing colonies) are cut out and placed on slides, with the colonies uppermost.
c) Stain-coated glass coverslips are applied to each agar block, with the stain face down. The glass should extend beyond the agar.
d) The space between slide and coverslip is filled with molten paraffin wax containing 10% yellow, soft paraffin. Upon cooling, the paraffin seals the preparation and permits oil immersion examination without displacing the coverslip.
e) Staining normally takes a few minutes, but it is advisable to wait 10–15 minutes before examining at 16 or 40×.
Note: If the agar is too thick or too opaque, it should first be pared by using a razor blade. The stain may be diluted if the agar takes up too much stain.

In either procedure, the typical structure of mycoplasma (or acholeplasma) colonies can be recognized: a dense, intensely stained center, a granular structure becoming thinner toward the edge, and a finely serrated border. Colonies of bacteria have a well-differentiated structure, often intensely and uniformly stained.

Suspicious mycoplasma cultures should also be checked for L-forms (spheroplasts and protoplasts of bacteria) by omission of penicillin from the media, which allows original bacteria to regain their shape. The organism should be purified by colony pick and allowed to grow in agar with bacterial inhibitors (thallium acetate and penicillin). After 3 subcultures, inhibitors should be omitted to check for L-forms.

Identification of M. mycoides

In the fluorescent antibody method, colonies on agar are identified as *M. mycoides* by staining with a positive reference fluorescein isothiocyanate (FITC) conjugate antiserum.[27,33] Growth and metabolic inhibition tests with known reference diagnostic sera may also be used.[5] Growth characteristics give additional support, as do fermentation of glucose, reduction of tetrazolium salt, and little or no proteolytic activity.

Serologic Diagnosis[13]

Detection of circulating antigen (galactan) may be achieved by an agar gel immunodiffusion test. The specific antigen galactan occurs on the surface of *M. mycoides* in the early stages of infection and is readily detected for 6–10 weeks after onset. It is widely distributed (in the blood, serum, lymph, pericardial fluid, and urine), but in chronic carriers, its frequency of detection drops sharply.

For detection of antibodies in individual sera, the complement fixation (CF)[3,9] test has been the most reliable, since it yields positive reactions from a greater proportion of cattle at different stages of infection than any other single test.[3,12,20] The CF test is not capable of detecting incubating or early acute cases, but does detect infected animals with lung sequestra. In chronic cases, large sequestra enclosed by a thick, fibrous connective tissue wall may not stimulate production of sufficient antibody, which leads to an occasional false negative result. Experimentally, positive results always indicate the presence of sequestra in the lung; negative results always indicate their absence. The test detects antibody from about 10 days after the onset of the disease. During the clinical stage of the disease, practically no sick animal gives a negative result. In vaccinated animals, the CF test can be positive for 3–6 months after vaccination. Therefore, a presumptive diagnosis of CBPP cannot be made in countries where vaccination of cattle is practiced.

The slide agglutination blood test is considerably less reliable than the slide agglutination serum test for serological diagnosis of CBPP.[12,21]

Growth and metabolic inhibition tests[5] are easy to perform and are accurate for detecting antibodies. The growth inhibition test is the method of choice in wildlife surveys for CBPP infection because it is more specific (although less sensitive) than the CF test.

The enzyme-linked immunosorbent assay (ELISA)[30] is very sensitive and detects all antibodies to *M. mycoides* whereas the CF test detects mainly the anti-galactan antibodies. There is a good correlation between the results of the two techniques.

Passive hemagglutination[4,6] and latex particle agglutination[31] tests have been used to some extent.

No test is capable of detecting CBPP-infected animals at every stage of the disease. However, the CF test has proven valuable in eradication and control of CBPP. An ideal test would detect all acute, chronic, and carrier CBPP-infected animals; could be used on a large scale in the field; would show negligible false-positive or -negative results; and would differentiate between infected and vaccinated animals. An accurate intradermal allergic test might meet these criteria, however, the necessity to read the delayed skin reaction up to 48 hours later is a definite handicap of the test.[11,36,41]

Acute CBPP cannot be confirmed by clinical signs alone because it is impossible to differentiate the disease clinically from other forms of pneumonia. At necropsy, the lesions should be highly suggestive of CBPP. Diagnosis must be confirmed by isolation and identification of *M. mycoides* by adding 10 ml of blood to 90 ml of liquid mycoplasma media, or culturing mycoplasma from aseptically collected exudate or affected lung tissue.

False positive CF test results may be due to certain bacteria[14,15] and *M. mycoides* subsp. *capri.*[7] Pulmonary pasteurellosis may simulate CBPP at necropsy but can be differentiated by observing the typical bipolar-staining organism in methylene blue or Giemsa-stained blood or infected lung smears.

Typical "marbling" and sequestral-type lesions are definitely highly suggestive of CBPP. Lung lesions or pleural exudate can be aseptically collected for culture examination or for use in direct agar gel immunodiffusion tests.[12]

Serological or biological confirmation of *M. mycoides* in the United States can only be accomplished at the Foreign Animal Disease Diagnostic Laboratory (FADDL). Samples of viable mycoplasma isolates or lung lesion material from suspicious CBPP animals should be sent to FADDL through the veterinarian in charge of the area in question.

Epidemiology

CBPP was once widespread in Africa, Europe, the United States, and some parts of Asia. The disease was eradicated from the United States in 1892 and Australia in 1973. All countries of Europe have been free of CBPP since the beginning of the 20th century, but recently the disease has been reported in Spain and Portugal. While widespread in many African countries and a few regions of Asia, it has never been reported in Madagascar or South America.

M. mycoides survives 2–3 days in the tropics, but 1–3 weeks in temperate regions. It survives 2 minutes at 60°C, 1 hour at 56°C, and 6 hours at 45°C. However, normal saline inactivates *M. mycoides* in 2 hours at 45°C and in less than a minute at 47°C.[29] Ultraviolet radiation inactivates cultures within a few minutes (loss of 10^6 log_{10} in 15 minutes).

CBPP is inactivated by wetting agents like saponin, digitonin, bile, and bile salts (sodium deoxycholate, at a concentration $3 \times 10^{-5}M$). Ordinary antiseptics also inactivate *M. mycoides:* 1% phenol solution (3 minutes), 0.5% formaldehyde solution (30 seconds), 0.01% mercuric chloride (1 minute), calcium hydroxide (less than 5 minutes), ether (less than 5 minutes) and 0.004% mercurochrome (60 minutes). Alcohol and boric acid have no effect.

Individual cattle differ in their susceptibility to CBPP. Some develop severe "Willem's reaction" following subcutaneous inoculation of *M. mycoides,* while others show no signs. Not all infected cattle become ill, and an animal serologically positive by the CF test may not show visible lung lesions.[39] Natural resistance of cattle to CBPP is unpredictable. Different cattle breeds vary in their resistance and susceptibility. Age is a determining factor, as calves are highly susceptible while yearlings are more resistant. Cattle are again more susceptible in old age. Beef steers are more resistant than dairy cows, and a possible difference exists in susceptibility of native zebu and exotic cattle.[17,26]

Infection can be experimentally produced by endobronchial or intravenous inoculation of a viable *M. mycoides* culture. Infection can not result when susceptible animals are introduced into areas previously occupied by infected stock, nor can contaminated feed spread the disease. Also, cattle do not develop CBPP when exposed to diseased lungs or animals which have died from the disease. Exposure via the conjunctival sac does not produce CBPP. Infection of susceptible cattle normally follows inhalation of infected droplets expelled by the coughing of an infected animal. Aerosol droplets from infected cattle can be carried 20 m or more by air currents to susceptible cattle. The way an animal with a viable sequestrum infects contact cattle is not precisely known; however, it is thought that discharge of infected material through a bronchus can lead to spread of infection. Another mode of spread may be via urine.[28]

Young calves are usually not important reservoirs of infection. More often they develop arthritic rather than pulmonary forms, and therefore are less likely to disseminate infections. There is evidence that *M. mycoides* may cross the placental barrier and infect the fetus.[40]

Factors influencing rate of spread of infection include proximity of animals, intensity of infection, level of susceptibility of individual animals, and stress conditions. Recovery from an outbreak gives a substantial degree of resistance to survivors. However, calves born after an outbreak may constitute a reservoir of infection. Climate and season have no direct effect on the disease, but contribute to spread. Also, spread of the disease is directly related to the type of husbandry used. During dry weather, the infective aerosols from infected cattle evaporate rapidly and the pathogen is inactivated by ultraviolet rays of the sun, thus diminishing the risk of spread. This is not the case in rainy seasons and cold weather, which may also lower the resistance of individual animals.

Immunity

The natural resistance of cattle is important when using or testing vaccines. Vaccines produced from live *M. mycoides* are superior to vaccines prepared with inactivated organisms.[34]

Animals recovered from CBPP possess a reliable immunity to reinfection. It is known that protection to CBPP coincides with the presence of mycoplasmas in ganglionic sites (nerve ganglion and organic lymph nodes).[24] For vaccination to be effective, it is very important that the organism multiply within the body.

Vaccines are prepared from the T_1 strain in East Africa, strain KH_3J (now extensively used in West Central Africa and Sudan[25]), and strain V_5 in Australia. Vaccination is generally believed to give good immunity for 2 or more years.[18] Vaccines are inoculated subcutaneously in the side of the neck, into the muzzle, behind the shoulder, or into the tail-tip. The tail-tip route is preferred because of its ease of inoculation, and less serious problems result if a severe reaction occurs.

Strain T_1 vaccine is produced from broth culture using the 44th egg passage strain ($T_1/44$) and strain T_1-SR (Maisons-Alfort) obtained after three passages in the presence of an increasing concentration of streptomycin. The vaccine must have a minimum titer of 5×10^8 viable organisms per ml; each 0.5 ml of the vaccine must contain 10^7 viable organisms. It produces variable local reactions and excellent immunity. Mycoplasma may be isolated from the blood for a brief period following vaccination. Antigen can be demonstrated in various tissues up to 200 days following vaccination, and 30–100% of vaccinates seroconvert, but the antibody is nondetectable within 60 days. Only 1% of vaccinated zebu show any vaccine reaction, whereas 25% of vaccinated cattle develop a reaction of severe necrosis, ulceration, and general infection.

Strain KH_3J originated in the Sudan. The vaccine is prepared in broth culture using the 88th egg passage. Both large and small colonies grow on agar plates and the larger resembles *M. mycoides* colonies. Inoculation does not produce local "Willem's reactions," but organisms can be isolated from the blood for a short time and antigen is detected from lymph nodes and lung tissue for 2 months. Seroconversion is rare.

Strain KH₃J-SR is a streptomycin-resistant strain that has been used in combination with a rinderpest vaccine for immunizing cattle.

Strain V₅ is an Australian vaccine produced after 85 passages.

Control

The "stamping out" method is preferred when infection is detected early, the extent of the outbreak is limited, and staff and finances are available. All cattle movements are stopped, all infected and possible contact cattle slaughtered, and compensation paid for destroyed animals. With large numbers of cattle, or when this method of control is economically infeasible, testing and slaughter may be necessary. Clinical cases and CF-positive reactors are slaughtered. All infected and contact herds must be isolated for several months, so it may be useful to combine testing and slaughter with vaccination of susceptible animals.

Another method of control is chemotherapy using a broad spectrum antibiotic. This is recommended only for control of severe reactions to vaccines, since its use on actual cases of CBPP could lead to a high incidence of carrier animals with sequestra in their lungs. In 1967 the Food and Agriculture Organization (FAO)/Office of International Epizootics (OIE)/ Organization of African Unity (OAU) panel unanimously opposed chemotherapeutic treatment of actual cases of CBPP and strongly recommended that mass drug or antibiotic treatment of CBPP be discouraged.[10]

References

1. Brown RD: 1963, Endobronchial inoculation of cattle with various strains of *Mycoplasma mycoides* and the effects of stress. Res Vet Sci 5:393–404.

2. Bygrave AC, Moulton JE, Shifrine M: 1988, Clinical, serological and pathological findings in an outbreak of contagious bovine pleuropneumonia. Bull Epizoot Dis Afr 16(1):21–46.

3. Campbell AD, Turner AW: 1953, Studies on contagious pleuropneumonia of cattle. IV. An improved complement fixation test. Aust Vet J 29:154–163.

4. Chima JC, Onoviran O, Pam C: 1984, An evaluation of the passive hemagglutination and complement fixation test in the diagnosis of contagious bovine pleuropneumonia, 4th International Congress of the International Organization of Mycoplasmology, Tokyo, Japan, 1982 Yale J Biol Med 57(6):905–906.

5. Clyde WA Jr: 1964, Mycoplasma species identification based upon growth inhibition by specific antisera. J Immunol 92:958–965.

6. Cottew GS: 1960, Indirect hemagglutination and hemagglutination inhibition with *Mycoplasma mycoides*. Aust Vet J 36:54–56.

7. Cottew GS, Yeats FR: 1978, Subdivision of *Mycoplasma mycoides* subsp. *mycoides* from cattle and goats into two types. Aust Vet J 54:293–296.

8. Daubney R: 1935, Contagious bovine pleuropneumonia. Note on experimental reproduction and infection by contact. J Comp Pathol 48:83–96.

9. Etheridge JR, Cottew GS, Lloyd LC: 1976, Studies on the origin of false positive reactions to the complement fixation test for contagious bovine pleuropneumonia. Aust Vet J 52:299–304.

10. FAO: 1967, Report of the third meeting of the FAO/OIE/OAU expert panel on contagious bovine pleuropneumonia, Khartoum, Sudan, 12–15 February.

11. Gourlay RN: 1962, An intradermal reaction produced by an extract of *Mycoplasma mycoides*. Vet Rec 74:1321.

12. Gourlay RN: 1965, Comparison between some diagnostic tests for contagious bovine pleuropneumonia. J Comp Path 75:375–380.

13. Gourlay RN: 1983, Serological tests for the diagnosis and control of contagious bovine pleuropneumonia and other infections with *Mycoplasma mycoides*. A Seminar in the CEC Program of Coordination of Research on Animal Pathology, Brussels, 16–17 June, pp. 27–32.

14. Gourlay RN, Howard CJ: 1979, Bovine mycoplasmas. In: The Mycoplasmas. Eds. Tully JG and Whitcomb RF, pp. 49–102. Academic Press, London.

15. Hayflick L: 1969, The *Mycoplasmatales* and the L-phase of bacteria, p. 750. North Holland Publishing Co., Amsterdam.

16. Hudson JR: 1971, Contagious bovine pleuropneumonia. Food and Agriculture Organization of the United Nations, Rome. FAO Agricultural Studies, No. 86.

17. Hudson JR: 1968, Contagious bovine pleuropneumonia experiments on the susceptibility and protection by vaccination of different types of cattle. Aust Vet J 44:83–89.

18. Hudson JR, Turner AW: 1963, Contagious bovine pleuropneumonia: A comparison of the efficacy of two types of vaccine. Aust Vet J 39(10):373–385.

19. Hyslop N: 1958, The adaption of *Asterococcus mycoides* of rodents. J Path & Bact 75:189.

20. Karst O: 1970, Contagious bovine pleuropneumonia: A plate complement fixation test employed at the Federal Department of Veterinary Research. Bull Epizoot Dis Afr 18:5–11.

21. Lindley EP: 1958, The rapid slide agglutination test in the control of contagious bovine pleuropneumonia in Nigeria. Bull Epizoot Dis Afr 6:369–371.

22. Lindley EP: 1973, Control measures against bovine pleuropneumonia in Ivory Coast. World Animal Review 6:1–5.

23. Martel JL, Belli P, Perrin M, Dannacher G, Poumarat F: 1958, La péripneumonie bovine contagieuse. In: pathologic respiratoire des bovine. Recl Med Vet 161(12):1105–1113.

24. Masiga WN, Mugera GM: 1973, Fate of the T strain of *Mycoplasma mycoides* in cattle following vaccination. J Comp Path 83(4):473–479.

25. Masiga WN, Read WCS: 1972, Comparative susceptibility of *Bos taurus* to contagious bovine pleuropneumonia, and the efficacy of the T_1 broth culture vaccine. Vet Rec 90:499–502.

26. Masiga WN, Stone SS: 1968, Fluorescent antibody and agar gel diffusion techniques to detect *Mycoplasma mycoides* in fresh and formalin-fixed lung lesions of cattle. Bull Epizoot Dis Afr 16(4):399–404.

27. Masiga WN, Stone SS: 1968, Application of a fluorescent antibody technique for the detection of *Mycoplasma mycoides* antigen and antibody. J of Bact 96(1):1867–1869.

28. Masiga WN, Windsor RS, Read WCS: 1972, A new mode of spread of contagious bovine pleuropneumonia. Vet Rec 90:247–248.

29. Mornet P, Orue J, Diagne L: 1949, Étude du phénomène de Willems dans la péripneumonie bovine. Bull Serv Elev AOF, 2(2–3):7–14.

30. Oroviran O, Taylor-Robinson D: 1979, Detection of antibody against *Mycoplasma*

mycoides subsp. *mycoides* in cattle by an enzyme-linked immunosorbent assay. Vet Rec 105:165–167.

31. Perreau P: 1963, Emploi de particules de latex dans la serologie de la péripneumonie des bovides. Rev Elev Med Vet Pays Trop 16(3):299–304.

32. Razin S, Freundt EA: 1984, Class 1. Mollicutes: Edward and Freundt 1967, 267AL Bergey's Manual of Systemic Bacteriology, ed. Krieg NR and Holt JG. Vol. I:763–765.

33. Rosendal S, Black FT: 1972, Direct and indirect immunofluorescence of unfixed and fixed colonies. Acta Path Microbiol Scand 80:615–622.

34. Shifrine M, Beech J: 1968, Preliminary studies on living culture and inactivated vaccines against contagious bovine pleuropneumonia. Bull Epizoot Dis Afr 16(1):47–52.

35. Shifrine M, Domermuth CH: 1967, Contagious bovine pleuropneumonia in wildlife. Bull Epizoot Dis Afr 15:319–322.

36. Shifrine M, Gourlay RN: 1965, The immediate type allergic skin reaction in contagious bovine pleuropneumonia. J Comp Path 75:381–385.

37. Shifrine M, Moulton JE: 1968, Infection of cattle with *Mycoplasma mycoides* by nasal installation. J Comp Path 78:383–386.

38. Smith GR: 1965, Infection of small laboratory animals with *Mycoplasma mycoides* var *capri* and *Mycoplasma mycoides* var *mycoides*. Vet Rec 77(50):1527–1528.

39. Stone SS, Bygrave AC: 1968, Contagious bovine pleuropneumonia: Comparison of serological tests and post mortem observations in cattle with resolving lung lesions. Bull Epizoot Dis Afr 16(4):399–404.

40. Stone SS, Masiga WN, Read WCS: 1969, *Mycoplasma mycoides* transplacental transfer in cattle. Res Vet Sci 10:368–372.

41. Windsor RS, Masiga WN, Boarer CDH: 1974, A single comparative intradermal test for the diagnosis of contagious bovine pleuropneumonia. Res Vet Sci 17:5–23.

Mycoplasmas of the Bovine Respiratory Tract

L. H. LAUERMAN

The severity of mycoplasma pneumonia is dramatically exhibited in contagious bovine pleuropneumonia (CBPP). The other mycoplasmas that infect the bovine respiratory tract produce a much less severe respiratory disease. The bovine mycoplasmas produce three main types of respiratory lesions. A serofibrinous pleuropneumonia is produced by *Mycoplasma mycoides* subsp. *mycoides* (see section above). The second type of respiratory lesion is produced by *M. bovis* and observed histologically as focal areas of coagulative necrosis surrounded by mononuclear cells and suppurative bronchitis with varying degrees of lymphoreticular hyperplasia (cuffing).[15,16,18,21] This lesion has been used to presumptively diagnose *M. bovis* on histological grounds in field cases of calf pneumonia. It is then confirmed by immunoperoxidase labeling on formalin-fixed paraffin-wax-embedded tissue.[29] The third type of respiratory lesion is an alveolitis, produced by *M. dispar*, in which neutrophils, macrophages, and edema fluid accumulate in the alveolar walls and spaces.[11,14,15] *M. dispar* has also been reported to produce histopathological lesions consisting of mononuclear cell infiltration, cuffing, catarrhal bronchiolitis, and atelectasis.[19] Field cases of subclinical pneumonia caused by *M. dispar* have been described with similar lesions.[25,28]

Gnotobiotic calves have been used effectively to evaluate the pathogenicity of various species of mycoplasmas isolated from the bovine respiratory tract.[12–16,18,19] Clinical signs of pneumonia were not present, but gross pneumonic lesions were observed in gnotobiotic calves inoculated with *M. bovis, M. dispar*, or *Ureaplasma* spp. *M. bovigenitalium* is rarely isolated from the bovine respiratory tract but produces a subclinical cuffing-type pneumonia in gnotobiotic calves.[13,14] Six other *Mycoplasma* and *Acholeplasma* species that have been isolated from the bovine respiratory tract did not induce pneumonia in gnotobiotic calves: *M. alkalescens, M. arginini, M. bovirhinis, M. canadense, A. axanthum*, and *A. modicum*.[14]

The preceding paragraphs describe lesions produced by infection initiated by individual species of mycoplasma. Bovine respiratory disease is considered of multiple etiology, and more recent reports describe experimental infections with mycoplasma and other infectious agents.[16,18,19,30] Gnotobiotic calves have been inoculated intranasally with *M. bovis* or *Pasteurella haemolytica* or both combined, and a severe disease was seen with the combined infection, suggestive of a synergistic reaction. The lung lesions in all calves with macroscopic pneumonia, whether inoculated with a single or combined agent, were histologically described as acute exudative pneumonia and only varied in extent and severity of lesions.[16,18] Mixed infections of *M. dispar* and *P. haemolytica* have been demonstrated in field cases of calf pneumonia.[28] Combined infections of *M. bovis* and respiratory syncytial virus in gnotobiotic calves were described.[29] The dual infection did not enhance the lesions observed. *M. bovis* was frequently isolated in large numbers from the upper and lower respiratory tract of cattle in an outbreak of infectious bovine rhinotracheitis.[2]

Cultural Examination

Specimens submitted to the laboratory for culture should be moist swabs (not submerged in liquid), with the samples being collected from deep within the nasal passage, as well as from the tonsils, trachea, and bronchi. Pediatric swabs may be used to reach into the bronchi. Tracheal and bronchial washes are used for culture, as well as sections of diseased lung. Refrigerate the samples on wet ice during transit to the laboratory.

On arrival, specimens should be promptly inoculated onto two types of freshly prepared solid media (Friis', Table 5.1 and Hayflick's, Addendum I) and incubated at 37°C in a high-humidity CO_2 incubator. Swabs are immersed in broth and vigorously twisted to suspend the mycoplasma, tissue fluids, and cell debris in the broth medium. Three 10-fold dilutions are made in both types of freshly prepared broth from the swab suspension and the tracheal and bronchial washings. Dilutions of macerated lung tissue are made to 10^{-9}. The specimen dilutions are incubated at 37°C for 2–3 days and passaged on agar media, as well as subpassaged in broth. *M. bovis* is easy to isolate in comparison to *M. dispar*, which is best isolated from broth cultures after several subpassages before attempting to grow it on agar. Normal calves generally have low levels of mixed mycoplasma flora in the nasal cavity (*M. bovirhinis, M. bovis, M. dispar, M. bovoculi, U. diversum, Acholeplasma, M. bovigenitalium*), whereas diseased calves have high levels of *M. bovis, M. dispar,* and/or *U. diversum,* with low levels of the other species.[14,15]

Rapid identification of the mixed colonies of mycoplasma on the original agar plate is performed by the direct immunofluorescent (IF) test (see Chapter 3).[1,9] Briefly, mycoplasma colonies on agar medium are enclosed with a circular plastic ring to form a well, covered with a drop of specific antibody conjugated with fluorescein isothiocyanate, incubated at 37°C in a humidified chamber for 30 minutes, and washed with phosphate-buffered saline (PBS) at pH 7.4. The reacted colonies are observed for fluorescence with a microscope using ultraviolet light. Subcultures from broth cultures onto agar are reacted by the IF test to confirm the results of the original agar plate.

Final identification is made on pure cultures, which are obtained by triple-cloning each colony isolated from the samples, then performing biochemical and serological tests (see Chapter 3). Resistance to digitonin differentiates the acholeplasmas from mycoplasmas and ureaplasmas, which are sensitive to digitonin. The acholeplasmas are speciated using the IF test. The ureaplasmas are urease-positive, which differentiates them from the mycoplasmas. The ureaplasmas are further identified using the IF test.[9] Six biochemical tests are routinely used to aid in identification of mycoplasma isolates: catabolism of arginine and glucose, phosphatase activity, digestion of coagulated horse serum, and reduction of tetrazolium chloride under aerobic and anaerobic conditions (Table 5.2). The mycoplasma isolates are further identified using three serological tests (IF, growth inhibition, and growth precipitation) with species-specific antisera.[6,8,9]

If additional tests are required for identification, turn first to Bergey's Manual of Systematic Bacteriology,[23] then consider electrophoretic analysis

Table 5.1. Friis' medium modified[10,11]

A. 2× Friis
1. Combine the following ingredients:
brain heart infusion (Difco)	49.29 g
PPLO w/o crystal violet (Difco)	52.29 g
Hank's balanced salt solution (Difco)	3.00 bottles
1% herring sperm DNA (Sigma)	16.00 ml
L-arginine (Sigma)	0.45 g
L-glutamine (Sigma)	0.68 g
1% phenol red	2.50 ml
distilled H_2O	3734.00 ml
2. Prepare 1% cysteine (Sigma). — 15.00 ml
3. Add NAD to the 1% cysteine. — 0.75 g
4. Add NAD-cysteine solution to mixture prepared in step 1.
5. Filter through a 0.22 μm filter to sterilize (requires prefiltration first).
6. Store at 4°C.

B. Yeast extract preparation
1. Bring 1816 ml distilled H_2O to 80°C on a stir plate.
2. Add 50 ml 6N HCL (pH should be 4.5 *after* yeast is added).
3. Slowly add 454 g brewers' yeast (Fleischmann's type 20–40) while stirring.
4. Check pH and adjust to 4.5.
5. Bring mixture to 80°C and hold at 80°C for 20 minutes.
6. Centrifuge yeast cells to remove them.
7. Filter through a 0.22μm filter to sterilize (requires prefiltration).
8. Store at −70°C.

C. Friis' broth
1. Add aseptically:
2× Friis	50 ml
fetal calf serum	20 ml
yeast extract	2 ml
2% bacitracin	1 ml
1% thallium acetate	1 ml
distilled H_2O (sterile)	25 ml
2. Adjust pH to 7.5 with sterile 1N NaOH.
3. Store at 4°C.

D. Friis' agar
1. Combine the following ingredients:
Noble agar	4.80 g
DEAE dextran (Sigma)	0.04 g
distilled H_2O	100.00 ml
2. Autoclave 15 minutes and cool to 56°C.
3. In another bottle combine aseptically:
2× Friis	200 ml
fetal calf serum	80 ml
yeast extract	8 ml
2% bacitracin	4 ml
1% thallium acetate	4 ml
7.5% sodium bicarbonate	4 ml
4. Adjust the pH to 7.5 with sterile 1N NaOH and warm to 45°C.
5. Add warm mixture from step 3 to cooled agar mixture in step 1 and pour into petri plates.

of proteins by SDS-PAGE; two-dimensional electrophoresis, and immunoblotting;[3,4,26] detection of enzymes, such as ornithine transcarbamylase;[27] determination of G + C contents of DNA; oligonucleotide probes;[5,24] or DNA amplification using polymerase chain reaction (PCR) for *M.*

Table 5.2.   Biochemical parameters for bovine *Mycoplasma* species or serogroups[7,23]

Species or Serogroup	Arg	Glu	Phos	S/D	Tetra
M. alkalescens	+	−	+	−	−/−
M. arginini	+	−	−	−	−/+
M. bovigenitalium	−	−	+	−	−/+
M. bovirhinis	−	+	−	−	+/+
M. bovis	−	−	+	−	+/+
M. bovoculi	−	+	−	−	+/+
M. canadense	+	−	w	−	−/+
M. dispar	−	+	−	−	+/+
M. mycoides subsp. mycoides	−	+	−	+/w	+/+
Group 7 of Leach	−	+	−	+	+/+

Note: Arg = arginine hydrolysis; Glu = glucose fermentation; Phos = phosphatase activity; S/D = serum digestion; Tetra = tetrazolium chloride reduction (aerobic/anaerobic); − = negative; + = positive; w = weak positive.

bovis.[17] A PCR assay for detection of mycoplasmas in general has recently been described utilizing 16S rRNA gene sequence data, and species may be identified by selecting probes from the variable regions of the amplicon.[31] Techniques using DNA probes and/or PCR DNA amplification should soon be available for routine identification of a number of mycoplasmas.

Direct examination of diseased lung tissue using the IF test on frozen lung sections is reported to be a rapid diagnostic method for bovine mycoplasmas.[22] The correlation demonstrated between this test and isolation was 82%. Mycoplasmas were detected in 9 of the 96 positive cases by the IF test alone. It appears that cryostat sectioning of diseased lung tissue will provide a rapid (1 day) diagnosis of specific mycoplasma infection.

Various serological tests have been used to detect and quantitate antibodies to mycoplasmas. A serological response to *M. bovis* invariably follows infection and has been detected by a variety of techniques, including indirect hemagglutination, single radial hemolysis, complement fixation, and enzyme immunoassay.[20] Antibodies to *M. dispar* have been demonstrated much less frequently than *M. bovis* because the former appears to be limited to the surface of the lung.[20] Antibodies to *M. dispar* can be demonstrated by single radial hemolysis and enzyme immunoassay.[20]

References

1. Al-Aubaidi JM, Fabricant J: 1971, The practical application of immunofluorescence (agar block technic) for the identification of *Mycoplasma*. Cornell Vet 61:519–542.
2. Allan EM, Pirie HM, Msolla PM, Selman IE, Wiseman A: 1980, The pathological features of severe cases of infectious bovine rhinotracheitis. Vet Rec 107:441–445.
3. Andersen H, Birkelund S, Christiansen G, Freundt EA: 1987, Electrophoretic analysis of proteins from *Mycoplasma hominis* strains detected by SDS-PAGE, two-dimensional gel electrophoresis and immunoblotting. J Gen Microbiol 133:181–191.

4. Andersen H, Christiansen G, Christiansen C: 1984, Electrophoretic analysis of proteins from *Mycoplasma capricolum* and related serotypes using extracts from intact cells and from minicells containing cloned mycoplasma DNA. J Gen Microbiol 130:1409–1418.

5. Christiansen C, Erno H: 1982, Classification of caprine strains by DNA hybridization. J Gen Microbiol 128:2523–2526.

6. Erno H, Peterslund K: 1983, Growth precipitation test: In: Methods in Mycoplasmology, Vol. 1. Ed. Razin S, Tully JG, pp. 489–492. Academic Press, London.

7. Erno H: 1987, Mycoplasmosis of ruminants: A general introduction. Rev Sci Tech Off Int Epizoot 6:553–563.

8. Freundt EA, Erno H, Lemcke RM: 1979, Identification of mycoplasma. In: Methods in Microbiology, Vol. 13. Eds. Bergan T, Norris JR, pp. 378–434. Academic Press, London.

9. Frey ML, Thomas GB, Hale PA: 1973, Recovery of and identification of mycoplasmas from animals. Ann NY Acad Sci 225:334–346.

10. Friis NF: 1975, Some recommendations concerning primary isolation of *Mycoplasma suipneumoniae* and *Mycoplasma flocculare*. Nord Vet Med 27:337–339.

11. Friis NF: 1980. *Mycoplasma dispar* as a causative agent in pneumonia of calves. Acta Vet Scand 21:34–42.

12. Gourlay RN, Thomas LH, Howard CJ: 1976, Pneumonia and arthritis in gnotobiotic calves following inoculation with *Mycoplasma bovis*. Vet Rec 98:506–507.

13. Gourlay RN, Howard CJ: 1978, Isolation and pathogenicity of mycoplasmas from the respiratory tract of calves. Curr Top Vet Med 3:295–304.

14. Gourlay RN, Howard CJ, Thomas LH, Wyld SG: 1979, Pathogenicity of some mycoplasmas and *Acholeplasma* species in the lungs of gnotobiotic calves. Res Vet Sci 27:233–237.

15. Gourlay RN, Howard CJ: 1982, Respiratory mycoplasmosis. Adv Vet Sci Comp Med 26:289–332.

16. Gourlay RN, Houghton SB: 1985, Experimental pneumonia in conventionally reared and gnotobiotic calves by dual infection with *Mycoplasma bovis* and *Pasteurella haemolytica*. Res Vet Sci 38:377–382.

17. Hotzel H: 1991, Personal communication. Jena, Germany.

18. Houghton SB, Gourlay RN: 1983, Synergism between *Mycoplasma bovis* and *Pasteurella haemolytica* in calf pneumonia. Vet Rec 113:41–42.

19. Howard CJ, Gourlay RN, Thomas LH, Stott EJ: 1976, Induction of pneumonia in gnotobiotic calves following inoculation of *Mycoplasma dispar* and ureaplasmas (T-mycoplasmas). Res Vet Sci 21:227–231.

20. Howard CJ: 1983, Mycoplasmas and bovine respiratory disease: Studies related to pathogenicity and the immune response – A selective review. Yale J Biol Med 56:789–797.

21. Jarrett WFH, McIntyre WIM, Urquhart GM: 1953, Recent work on husk: A preliminary report on an atypical pneumonia. Vet Rec 65:153–156.

22. Knudtson WU, Reed DE, Daniels G: 1986, Identification of Mycoplasmatales in pneumonic calf lungs. Vet Microbiol 11:79–91.

23. Krieg NR, Holt JG: 1984, Bergey's Manual of Systematic Bacteriology. Williams and Wilkins, Baltimore/London, Vol. 1, 9th edition.

24. Mattsson JG, Gersdorf H, Göbel UB, Johansson KE: 1991, Detection of *Mycoplasma bovis* and *Mycoplasma agalactiae* by oligonucleotide probes complementary to 16S rRNA. Molecular & Cellular Probes 5:27–35.

25. Pirie HM, Allan EM: 1975, Mycoplasmas and cuffing pneumonia in a group of calves. Vet Rec 97:345–349.

26. Rodwell AW: 1982, The protein fingerprints of mycoplasmas. Rev Infect Dis 4:S8–S17.

27. Salih MM, Erno H, Simonsen V: 1983, Electrophoretic analysis of isoenzymes of mycoplasma species. Acta Vet Scand 24:14–33.

28. St George TD, Horsfall N, Sullivan ND: 1973, A subclinical pneumonia of calves associated with *Mycoplasma dispar.* Aust Vet J 49:580–586.

29. Thomas LH, Howard CJ, Stott EJ, Parsons KR: 1986, *Mycoplasma bovis* infection in gnotobiotic calves and combined infection with respiratory syncytial virus. Vet Pathol 23:571–578.

30. Tinant MK, Bergland ME, Knudtson WU: 1979, Calf pneumonia associated with *Mycoplasma dispar* infection. J Am Vet Med Assoc 175:812–813.

31. van Kuppeveld FJM, van der Logt JTM, Angulo AF, van Zoest MJ, Quint WGV, Niesters HGM, Galama JMD, Melchers WJG: 1992, Genus- and species-specific identification of mycoplasmas by 16S rRNA amplification. Appl Environ Microbiol 58:2606–2615.

Mycoplasmas Associated with Bovine Genital Tract Infections

H. L. RUHNKE

Members of the Mycoplasmataceae family, including the genera *Mycoplasma, Ureaplasma,* and *Acholeplasma,* are common inhabitants of the genital tract of cattle. They are frequently isolated from apparently healthy animals, which would suggest that they are non-pathogenic.[4,5,13,18,20,21,32] However, there are strains of some species that have been shown to cause disease in susceptible animals, resulting in considerable losses in production.[7,10,11,12,18,32] The potential for international transmission of disease organisms with the transport of genetic material is an important consideration.[33]

Because of the number of mycoplasma species that may be recovered from the genital tract, speciation of isolates is important. *Ureaplasma* spp. can be identified on the primary plate by the production of brown colonies in the presence of manganese sulfate due to the reaction with the urease enzyme. *Mycoplasma* and *Acholeplasma* species can be identified by direct or indirect immunofluorescence on primary or first passage plates.

Ureaplasmosis

A number of studies since 1976 have shown that *Ureaplasma diversum* (formerly called T-strain mycoplasma) plays an important role in bovine reproductive failure.[7,9,10,11,27] Clinical signs include granular vulvitis, endometritis, salpingitis, abortion, infertility in the female, and seminovesiculitis in the male. Isolation of the organism from field cases has been followed by reproduction of each disease experimentally.[1-4,7-10,19,24]

Cows

Granular Vulvitis — Acute granular vulvitis is characterized by an inflamed hyperemic vulvar mucosa with small 1- to 2-mm raised granules usually clustered around the clitoris. A purulent discharge is present for 3–10 days and then the disease typically becomes chronic, with a gradual decline in the severity of the clinical signs. The organism may continue to be recovered from the vulva as long as 7 months after the acute onset of the disease. It may colonize the uterus at estrus but may be cleared within 7 days following infection, so uterine cultures may not give a true indication of disease due to ureaplasma.[7-10,27]

Infertility — During the acute phase, the organism has been shown to cause infertility, but the exact mechanism has not been determined. The chronic phase of the disease may also affect fertility if permanent damage has been caused to the endometrium and/or fallopian tubes.[9,19]

Embryo Transfer Fluids — *U. diversum* has been found in 10% of flush fluids. It is capable of adhering to the zona pellucida of the embryo and resists removal by washing.[6,10]

Abortion — *U. diversum* most commonly causes abortion in the last trimester, or calves may be stillborn or weak at birth and die shortly afterward with respiratory failure.[10,11,24,28] The organism may also be associated with early embryonic death and abortion in the first trimester. The cows are not ill, but the placental membranes are generally retained. Gross lesions in the placenta consist of marked thickening of large areas of the amnion and intercotyledonary zones in the chorioallantois. There may be foci of fibrin exudation and hemorrhage. Gross lesions have not been observed in the aborted fetus. Microscopic lesions are characteristic but not specific. Thickened regions of the placenta have diffuse fibrosis, a heavy infiltration of mononuclear cells, foci of necrosis, fibrin exudation, and mineralization. In the lung there is a diffuse alveolitis, and focal lymphocytic accumulations may be prominent around airways. The alveolitis is characterized by degeneration and necrosis of the alveolar epithelium, and there is infiltration of macrophages and granulocytes.

Bulls

Ureaplasmas are common contaminants of the prepuce and the distal urethra, having been reported in 29–100% of samples cultured. However, the presence of ureaplasma in these sites is generally not associated with clinical signs in the bull.[10,11,13,18] Contaminated raw semen (23–84% of bulls) is an important vehicle for transmission of ureaplasmas. Treatment of semen with the antibiotic combination gentamicin, lincospectin, and tylosin appears to control both mycoplasmas and ureaplasmas.[31,33] Seminovesiculitis has been reproduced experimentally[10] and ureaplasmas have been isolated from a few field cases.

No standardized serologic procedure for *Ureaplasma* diagnosis in cattle is currently available.

Specimen Collection and Handling

Isolation of ureaplasma in the genital tract of cows is most successful from cultures of vulvar swabs. Uterine swabs are less often culture-positive since the organism may remain in the uterus for only a short time.

Preputial swabs should be taken with a guarded unit to obtain the sample from as far into the cavity as possible. Semen should be collected following disinfection of the prepuce. Processed semen should be maintained in liquid nitrogen until ready to culture.

Preferred tissues from abortions are lung, caruncle, cotyledon, stomach content, and amniotic fluid. Fluids and tissues should be taken and handled as described in Chapter 2.

Ureaplasma Isolation

Media recommended for human ureaplasmas are usually not as satisfactory for primary isolation of animal ureaplasmas.[29,30] (See Addendum I for ureaplasma agar and broth.) To culture tissue, cut a small cube (2–3 cm). To sterilize, dip it in alcohol, ignite, and allow to burn off. Cut the cube in half with sterile scissors and rub the cut surface over one half of a plate of ureaplasma agar. Streak across the inoculum with a platinum loop. Mince tissue with sterile scissors (grinding is not recommended since inhibitory factors may be released), mix with 3–5 ml ureaplasma broth, and let stand a few minutes. Remove broth from tissues into a sterile tube and make four 10-fold dilutions. Dilutions may be plated immediately.

To culture fluids and swabs, inoculate swabs onto ureaplasma agar then swirl in ureaplasma broth. Discard the swab, and make four or more 10-fold dilutions. Inoculate a drop or two of fluids onto ureaplasma agar and streak out with a loop. Inoculate a broth tube with a 10% inoculum and make further 10-fold dilutions. Incubate broths aerobically and plates in an anaerobic jar with a H_2 plus CO_2 generator pack at 37°C.

Examine dilutions of ureaplasma broth in 18–24 hours for alkaline pH change and subculture to agar from tubes that have turned very slightly alkaline. Ureaplasmas are usually no longer viable when broth has become very alkaline. If there is no change in the broth, re-examine daily for 7 days before discarding as negative. Always confirm color change in broth by subculture to plates. Some arginine-positive mycoplasmas and some diphtheroids and yeasts may also cause an alkaline change in broth without turbidity.

Examine plates at 48 hours with a stereomicroscope (40× magnification) for typical brown colonies varying in size from small to large (the size of mycoplasma colonies). Plates are incubated 7–10 days before discarding as negative.

Mycoplasmosis

Mycoplasma bovigenitalium is a common mycoplasma species in genital tract disease[4,5,12,18,21,25,32] and has been shown to cause infertility, necrotizing endometritis, seminal vesiculitis, and impaired spermatozoa motility. *M. bovigenitalium* has also been isolated from aborted fetuses. Early studies linking this organism with granular vulvitis were carried out before recovery of *Ureaplasma* from the reproductive tract, and the significance of *M. bovigenitalium* in this syndrome remains to be determined.

M. bovis is a proven pathogen and has caused endometritis, salpingitis, oophoritis, abortion, and seminovesiculitis under experimental conditions,[12] but is infrequently isolated from the genital tract of cattle. It has been isolated occasionally from aborted fetuses, and one natural case of seminovesiculitis. It is an important cause of mastitis, arthritis, and pneumonia.

M. canadense is frequently isolated from the genital tract of bulls and sporadically from aborted fetuses. The organism also causes mastitis.[3,12]

Acholeplasma laidlawii is a frequent isolate from the bovine genital tract, often in association with other mycoplasmatales. It has not been shown to be the cause of any reproductive disease and is considered nonpathogenic.[12]

Other species that have been isolated from the reproductive tract but have not been proven to cause disease are *M. bovirhinis, M. alkalescens, M. arginini, M. verecundum, M. alvi, Mycoplasma* sp. Group 7, *A. axanthum,* and *A. oculi.*

Mycoplasma Isolation

Cultures for mycoplasmas should be made in duplicate using mycoplasma medium[14,15] (see Addendum I) containing horse serum or porcine serum, since some isolates grow better with porcine serum. Tissues, swabs, and fluids (except semen) are handled as for ureaplasmas. Special methods to isolate mycoplasmas from semen are described in Addendum I.

Incubate broths aerobically and plates in a moist atmosphere of 5–10% CO_2 in air at 37°C. Examine plates after 48 hours with a stereomicroscope for typical "fried egg" colonies, as described in Chapter 3. Subcultures from broth to agar medium should be made after 2, 4, and 7 days, even if no pH change has occurred. Some glycolytic mycoplasmas do not produce acid from glucose on primary culture and could be missed if pH is used as a marker of growth. As soon as colonies are seen, subcultures from plates can be made by cutting a small block of agar and rubbing it colony-side-down on a fresh plate. Single colonies may be subcultured to agar using a platinum loop; for transfer to broth the colony may be cut out with a fine-pointed scalpel.

Identification of Isolates

Ureaplasma is identified by the production of brown colonies on agar medium containing manganese sulfate, due to the deposition of manganese on the surface of the colony. The species isolated from cattle is *U. diversum*. Serotyping of isolates can be done by immunofluorescence on colonies grown on Howard's U4 agar[16,17] (see Addendum I). Most *U. diversum* isolates can be classified into serogroups A, B, and C, represented by type strains A417, D48, and T44, respectively. Typing sera are not available for distribution, so laboratories wishing to serotype *U. diversum* isolates must make their own antisera.[22,23]

Mycoplasma isolates can be identified directly from the primary agar plate or from an early subculture by immunofluorescence of colonies as described in Addendum I. Mixed cultures can be detected, and relative numbers of each species can be assessed using this technique.

Other techniques helpful in identifying isolates after cloning include growth inhibition using the well or disc method, metabolism inhibition in broth, glucose and arginine metabolism, phosphatase activity, sensitivity to digitonin, and digestion of serum or milk[22,23] as described in Chapter 3.

References

1. Ball HJ, McCaughey WJ, Mackie DP, Pearson GR: 1981, Experimental genital infection of heifers with ureaplasmas. Res Vet Sci 30:312–317.

2. Ball HJ, Armstrong D, Kennedy S, McCaughey WJ: 1987, Experimental intrauterine inoculation of cows at oestrus with a bovine ureaplasma strain. Irish Vet J 41:371–372.

3. Ball HJ, Armstrong D, McCaughey WJ, Kennedy S: 1987, Experimental intrauterine inoculation of cows at oestrus with *Mycoplasma canadense*. Vet Rec 120:370.

4. Ball HJ, Logan EF, Orr W: 1987, Isolation of mycoplasmas from bovine semen in Northern Ireland. Vet Rec 121:322–324.

5. Blom E, Friis NF, Ernø H: 1983, Mycoplasmas: Demonstration in semen and preputial washings from bulls. Acta Vet Scand 24:238–240.

6. Britton AP, Miller RB, Ruhnke HL, Johnson WH: 1988, The recovery of ureaplasmas from bovine embryos following *in vitro* exposure and ten washes. Theriogenology 30:997–1003.

7. Doig PA, Ruhnke HL, Mackay AL, Palmer NC: 1979, Bovine granular vulvitis associated with ureaplasma infection. Can Vet J 20:89–94.

8. Doig PA, Ruhnke HL, Palmer NC: 1980, Experimental bovine genital ureaplasmosis. I. Granular vulvitis following vulvar inoculation. Can J Comp Med 44:252–258.

9. Doig PA, Ruhnke HL, Palmer NC: 1980, Experimental bovine genital ureaplasmosis. II. Granular vulvitis, endometritis and salpingitis following uterine inoculation. Can J Comp Med 44:259–266.

10. Doig PA, Ruhnke HL, Waelchli-Suter R, Palmer NC, Miller RB: 1981, The role of ureaplasma infection in bovine reproductive disease. Compendium on Continuing Education 3: S324–S330.

11. Doig PA, Ruhnke HL: 1986, Effects of ureaplasma infection on bovine reproduction. In: Current Therapy in Theriogenology. Ed. Morrow DA, pp. 282–287. W. B. Saunders, Philadelphia.

12. Doig PA, Ruhnke HL: 1986, Effects of mycoplasma and acholeplasma infection on bovine reproduction. In: Current Therapy in Theriogenology. Ed. Morrow DA, pp. 288–291. W. B. Saunders, Philadelphia.

13. Fish NA, Rosendal S, Miller RB: 1985, The distribution of mycoplasmas and ureaplasmas in the genital tract of normal artificial insemination bulls. Can Vet J 26:13–15.

14. Gourlay RN, Howard CJ: 1983, Recovery and identification of bovine mycoplasmas. In: Methods in Mycoplasmology, Vol. 2, Diagnostic Mycoplasmology. Eds. Tully JG, Razin S, pp. 81–89. Academic Press, New York.

15. Hayflick L: 1965, Tissue cultures and mycoplasmas. Tex Rep Biol Med 23:285–303.

16. Howard CJ, Gourlay RN, Collins J: 1978, Serological studies with bovine ureaplasmas (T-Mycoplasmas). Int J Syst Bact 28: 473–477.

17. Howard CJ, Gourlay RN: 1981, Identification of ureaplasmas from cattle using antisera prepared in gnotobiotic calves. J Gen Microbiol 126:365–369.

18. Jurmanova K, Weznik Z, Cerna J, Mazurova J: 1983, Demonstration and role of mycoplasma and ureaplasma in bull semen and the control of mycoplasma infections in bulls. Arch Exp Veterinaermed 37:421–428.

19. Kreplin CMA, Ruhnke HL, Miller RB, Doig PA: 1987, The effect of intrauterine inoculation with *Ureaplasma diversum* on bovine fertility. Can J Vet Res 51:440–443.

20. Langford EV: 1974, Mycoplasma species recovered from the reproductive tracts of western Canadian cows. Can J Comp Med 39:133–138.

21. Langford EV: 1975, Mycoplasma recovered from bovine male and female genitalia and aborted feti. Proc 18th Annu Meet Am Assoc Vet Lab Diagn pp. 221–232.

22. Methods in Mycoplasmology, 1983, Vol. 1, Mycoplasma Characterization. Eds. Razin S, Tully JG, Academic Press, New York.

23. Methods in Mycoplasmology, 1983, Vol. 2, Diagnostic Mycoplasmology. Eds. Tully JG, Razin S, Academic Press, New York.

24. Miller RB, Ruhnke HL, Doig PA, Poitras BJ, Palmer NC: 1983, The effects of *Ureaplasma diversum* inoculated into the amniotic cavity in cows. Theriogenology 20:367–374.

25. Panangala VS, Winter AJ, Wijesinha MS, Foote RH: 1981, Decreased motility of bull spermatozoa caused by *Mycoplasma bovigenitalium*. Am J Vet Res 42:2090–2093.

26. Rosendal S, Black FT: 1972, Direct and indirect immunofluorescence of unfixed and fixed mycoplasma colonies. Acta Path Microbiol Scand B 80:615.

27. Ruhnke HL, Doig PA, Mackay AL, Gagnon A, Kierstead M: 1978, Isolation of ureaplasma from bovine granular vulvitis. Can J Comp Med 42:151–155.

28. Ruhnke HL, Palmer NC, Doig PA, Miller RB: 1984, Bovine abortion and neonatal death associated with *Ureaplasma diversum*. Theriogenology 21:295–301.

29. Shepard MC, Lunceford CD: 1976, Differential agar medium (A7) for identification of *Ureaplasma urealyticum* (Human T Mycoplasmas) in primary cultures of clinical material. J Clin Microbiol 3:613–625.

30. Shepard MC: 1983, Culture media for ureaplasmas. In: Methods in Mycoplasmology, Vol. 1, Mycoplasma Characterization. Eds. Razin S, Tully JG, pp. 137–146. Academic Press, New York.

31. Shin SJ, Lein DH, Patten VH, Ruhnke HL: 1988, A new antibiotic combination for frozen bovine semen. 1. Control of Mycoplasmas, Ureaplasmas, *Campylobacter fetus* subsp. *venerealis* and *Haemophilus somnus*. Theriogenology 29:577–591.

32. Trichard CJV, Jacobsz EP: 1985, Mycoplasmas recovered from bovine genitalia, aborted foetuses and placentas in the Republic of South Africa. Onderstepoort J Vet Res 52:105–110.

33. Truscott RB, Ruhnke HL: 1984, Control of mycoplasma and ureaplasma in semen. Proc Int Symp, Microbiological Tests for the International Exchange of Animal Genetic Material. Ed. Stalheim OHV, pp. 50–64. Am Assoc Vet Lab Diag Suppl.

Mycoplasmas and Bovine Mastitis

D. E. JASPER

Mastitis due to *Mycoplasma bovigenitalium* was first reported from England.[4,6,16,28] Soon thereafter a more severe form of mycoplasma mastitis was reported from Connecticut,[11] New York,[5] and California.[19] The latter outbreaks were due to a new species, first referred to as *M. agalactiae* subsp. *bovis,* also called *M. bovimastitidis,*[14] but later named *M. bovis.*[2] Mastitis due to *M. bovis* is found in all North American countries, most European countries, and some Asian countries.[4,16] Most mycoplasma mastitis outbreaks worldwide are due to *M. bovis;* however, a number of other mycoplasma species are also important causes.

A new species, *M. californicum,* has become the second most frequently found cause of mycoplasma mastitis in California.[18] It has also been reported from Ireland,[22] Scotland,[9] East Germany,[24] and other countries.[16] An outbreak of mastitis in dry cows due to *M. californicum* resulted in severe inflammation and many non-functioning quarters.[21]

Another mycoplasma, *M. canadense,* was described first in Canada,[20] but was previously recognized as a separate unknown species[7,8] in California, where it persists as an important mastitis pathogen. Less common causes of mastitis are *M. bovigenitalium* and *M. alkalescens.*[16] Isolation of *M. bovirhinis, M. arginini,* and *Acholeplasma laidlawii* are also reported,[16] the latter being of questionable pathogenicity and usually from contaminated samples. Even *M. capricolum,* hitherto considered an important pathogen only of goats, has also been associated with clinical mastitis in cows.[29] It is probable that other species may be involved at times.

Since mycoplasma mastitis can be a devastating disease on individual dairies, early diagnosis is very important. The mycoplasma should be identified by species in order to provide sound control recommendations.[16]

Clinical Signs

Mycoplasmal mastitis due to *M. bovis* is generally characterized by a sudden drop in milk production, often involving several or all four quarters.[15,16,19] In most cows the quarters are swollen. A day or so after production loss, some tannish discoloration appears in the milk and small flakes or a sandy sediment may be seen on the walls of collection tubes. Tannish discoloration and thickening follows with progression in many cases to a purulent exudate that may continue for weeks and possibly into the next lactation.[15,16,19] In endemic herds the inflammation may eventually be less intense. Duration of morbidity and extent of recovery vary.

Infected secretions may contain a high number of mycoplasma, and so are highly infectious. Shedding is common after clinical recovery and may be intermittent, rendering a single negative culture unreliable for determining shedder status. However, most recovered animals with normal secretions in the next lactation are not shedders.

Antibiotic or other specific therapy of mycoplasma mastitis has not been effective.[16]

Diagnosis and Identification

A positive diagnosis of mycoplasma mastitis is dependent upon isolation of mycoplasma from suspect milk (secretion) samples.[1] These may be quarter samples or composite samples. Tank milk samples are helpful for screening on a herd basis, although dilution could mask one or more shedders of low numbers. Milk samples for any cultural procedure must be collected with careful aseptic precautions.[23] Samples should be refrigerated or frozen during transit or storage prior to culture. Samples (and cultures) for long-term storage should be frozen, preferably at $-30°C$ or below to assure future viability.[16,19]

Samples are streaked in 0.01–0.05 ml amounts, or by use of cotton swabs, onto special mycoplasma agar plates, usually a modified Hayflick's medium[16,23] (see Addendum I). Sometimes, but not always, percent recoveries can be enhanced by pre-incubation of milk alone or with added broth.

L-forms of *Streptococcus agalactiae* or *Staphylococcus aureus* that appear very much like mycoplasma have been described.[27,30]

Identification of recovered mycoplasma is important to planning control procedures.[16] Although both biochemical and serologic methods are used, the best procedures are serologic.[3,10,16] We use the method described by Baas and Jasper[3] modified to the extent that 1 mg/L of thimerosal is added to the phosphate buffered saline and incubation time is lengthened to 75 minutes. Staining and washing are done within 1-cm-diameter cylinders that are pressed into the agar on the plates before the round agar blocks are removed to slides for reading.

In our experience, an immunoperoxidase test done on colonies using filter paper[12] has given excellent results, is easy to perform, and does not require fluorescence microscopy. An immunobinding test for use directly on suspect milk or culture for detection and/or identification has also been shown to recognize 5×10^3 or more organisms/ml.[13]

Prevention and Control

The most likely source of new mycoplasma infection in clean herds is the introduction of infected cows. Therefore, bulk tank milk from all herds of origin, especially those in endemic areas, should be cultured prior to purchase. Further assurance is gained if composite milk from individual animals is cultured prior to their entry into milking strings. It is best to confine purchases to herds known to be free of mycoplasma mastitis. We have known several instances of dairymen culling infected cows, then purchasing infected replacements.

Heifers sometimes calve with mycoplasma mastitis, the source of which is not always known. Cows or heifers, especially those from areas endemic for mycoplasma mastitis, should be monitored carefully to avoid introduction of infection. Early detection in endemic areas is abetted by a regular program of culturing samples from all clinical cases of mastitis for mycoplasma, as well as for bacteria. Monthly cultures of bulk tank milk may also aid early detection, as will culture of all new cows of any age entering the milking strings.[16]

Once infection is detected in a herd, the first objective should be to protect non-infected cows. This requires herd cultures of composite milk samples from all cows in the herd, plus cultures from clinical cases of mastitis and all fresh or other cows entering the milking strings. Infected cows should be segregated and milked after the clean cow strings. It is probably best to segregate cows having *M. bovis* infection for life, or send them to slaughter. For other mycoplasma species, it appears that infections seldom persist into the following lactation. Cows with persistent severe mycoplasma mastitis of any kind are best not kept in the herd.

Management practices strongly influence the risk of first infection, rapidity of spread, and effectiveness of control procedures. Of first importance is milking sanitation. Careful pre-milking preparation and post-milking teat-dipping with a recognized teat dip is recommended.[4,17]

During outbreaks, milkers should wear rubber gloves, sanitizing both gloves and teat cups between cows. Backflush systems are believed to be helpful in reducing spread of mycoplasma infections.[16,19] Improper function of milking machines is also believed to be a factor in spread of infection.[16,19] Machine function and milking management should be checked carefully in outbreak situations, and any faults corrected.

Mycoplasma mastitis is frequently spread at times of lactation or dry-cow treatment or both. It is not uncommon for milking cows treated for bacterial mastitis to develop mycoplasma mastitis soon afterwards because of careless treatment procedures. Herd treatments, as for *Streptococcus agalactiae* infections, present an opportunity for widespread introduction of mycoplasma infections. Carelessness occurring in "hospital" strings often spreads mycoplasma infections. An especially dangerous practice is the housing of newly calved cows with mastitic cows in special strings, which should be avoided at all times. Mycoplasma mastitis resulting from unsanitary treatment procedures at drying-off usually becomes apparent upon freshening.[16]

Mycoplasma such as *M. bovis* or *M. bovigenitalium* may be carried in respiratory or genital tracts of apparently well cattle, possibly serving as a source of mammary infection to them or other cattle.[16] Mycoplasma survive for variable periods of time on teat skin[17] and in the environment, e.g., only 1–2 days on wood and steel but several weeks on straw, sponges, manure, or in drinking water.[16,25,26] More information is needed upon the role of fomites in the spread of mycoplasma mastitis. Calves drinking mycoplasma-infected milk become respiratory carriers. These infections may contribute to some later pneumonia problems, but their significance is not really known. They have not been shown to result in mycoplasma mastitis, but the possibility has not been excluded.

References

1. Al-Aubaidi JM, Fabricant J: 1968, Techniques for the isolation of mycoplasma from cattle. Cornell Vet 58:555–571.
2. Aska G, Erno H: 1976, Elevation of *Mycoplasma agalactiae,* subsp. *bovis* to species rank: *Mycoplasma bovis* (Hale et al.) comb. nov. Int J Syst Bacterial 26:323–325.
3. Baas EJ, Jasper DE: 1976, Agar block technique for identification of mycoplasmas by fluorescent antibody. Appl Microbiol 23:1097–1100.
4. Boughton E: 1979, *Mycoplasma bovis* mastitis. Vet Bull 49:377–387.
5. Carmichael LE, Guthrie RS, Fincher MG, Field LE, Johnson SD, Lindquist WE: 1963, Bovine mycoplasma mastitis. Proc US Livestock San Assoc, 67th Annu Meet:220–235.
6. Davidson I, Stuart P: 1960, Isolation of a mycoplasma-like organism from an outbreak of bovine mastitis. Vet Rec 72:766.
7. Dellinger JD, Jasper DE: 1972, Polyacrylamide-gel electrophoresis of cell proteins of mycoplasma isolated from cattle and horses. Am J Vet Res 33:769–775.
8. Dellinger JD, Jasper DE, Ilic M: 1977, Characterization studies on mycoplasmas isolated from bovine mastitis and the bovine respiratory tract. Cornell Vet 67:352–357.
9. Gibbs HA, Allan EM: 1986, Mycoplasma mastitis outbreak (correspondence). Vet Rec 118: 647.
10. Gourlay RN, Howard CJ: 1983, Recovery and identification of bovine mycoplasmas. In: Methods in Mycoplasmology, Vol. 2, Diagnostic Mycoplasmology. Eds. Tully JG, Razin S, Vol. II, pp. 81–89. Academic Press Inc., New York.
11. Hale HH, Helmboldt CF, Plastridge WN, Stula EF: 1962, Bovine mastitis caused by a mycoplasma species. Cornell Vet 52:582–591.
12. Imada Y, Uchida I, Hashimoto K: 1987, Rapid identification of mycoplasmas by indirect immunoperoxidase test using small square filter paper. J Clin Micro 25:17–21.
13. Infante F, Jasper DE, Stott JL, Cullor JS, Dellinger JD: 1990, Immunobinding assay for detection of *Mycoplasma bovis* in milk. Can J Vet Res 54:251–255.
14. Jain NC, Jasper DE, Dellinger JD: 1967, Cultural characters and serological relationships of some mycoplasmas isolated from bovine sources. J Gen Microbiol 49:401–410.
15. Jasper DE: 1979, Bovine mycoplasmal mastitis. J Am Vet Med Assoc 75:1072–1074.
16. Jasper DE: 1981, Bovine mycoplasmal mastitis. Adv Vet Sci Comp Med 25:121–159.
17. Jasper DE, Dellinger JD, Hakanson HD: 1976, Effectiveness of certain teat dips and sanitizers *in vitro* and on the skin against *Mycoplasma agalactiae* subsp. *bovis*. Cornell Vet 66:164–171.
18. Jasper DE, Dellinger JD, Rollins MH, Hakanson HD: 1979, Prevalence of mycoplasmal mastitis in California. Am J Vet Res 40:1043–1047.
19. Jasper DE, Jain NC, Brazil LH: 1966, Clinical and laboratory observations on bovine mastitis due to mycoplasma. J Am Vet Med Assoc 148:1017–1029.
20. Langford EV, Ruhnke HL, Onoviran O: 1976, *Mycoplasma canadense,* a new bovine species. Int J System Bact 26:212–219.

21. Mackie DP, Ball HJ: 1986, *Mycoplasma californicum* mastitis in the dry dairy cow. Vet Rec 199:350–351.

22. Mackie DP, Ball HJ, Logan EF: 1982, Isolation of *Mycoplasma californicum* from an outbreak of bovine mastitis and experimental reproduction of the disease. Vet Rec 110:578–580.

23. National Mastitis Council: Microbiological procedures for the diagnosis of bovine mastitis. National Mastitis Council, 1940 Wilson Blvd, Arlington, VA 22201.

24. Pfutzner H, Wehnert C, Leirer R: 1986, Untersuchen zur eutervirulenz von *Mycoplasma californicum*. Archiv fur Exper Vetmed 40:56–62.

25. Rinaldi A, Redaelli G, Nani S, Ruffo G, Socci A: 1972, Some observations on the epizootiology of mycoplasmic bovine mastitis. Proc International Meet Dis Cattle (7th) 552–558.

26. Ruffo G, Nani S, Podesta A: 1968, Survival of *Mycoplasma agalactiae* var. *bovis* in several materials and at different temperatures. Archiv Vet Ital 20:459–464.

27. Sears PM, Netherton BF, Merrill RB: 1987, Induction of L-form variants of *Staphylococcus aureus* obtained from milk samples from cows. J Am Vet Med Assoc 191:681–684.

28. Stuart P, Davidson I, Slavin G: 1963, Bovine mastitis caused by mycoplasma. Vet Rec 75:59–64.

29. Taoudi A, Kirchhoff H: 1986, Isolation of *Mycoplasma capricolum* from cows with mastitis. Vet Rec 119:247.

30. Wilson CD, Little TWA, Roberts DH, Hardwick AG: 1971, The isolation of L-forms of *Streptococcus agalactiae* from cases of bovine mastitis. Br Vet J 127:253–263.

CHAPTER 6

Porcine Mycoplasmas

C. H. ARMSTRONG

There are three species of mycoplasmas that cause diseases in swine: *Mycoplasma hyopneumoniae* (*suipneumoniae*)[12,13], *M. hyorhinis*[23] and *M. hyosynoviae*.[17] *M. flocculare,*[8,14] a very fastidious species, appears to be a common inhabitant of the porcine lung,[3] but is essentially non-pathogenic.[9,10] Several other species of Mollicutes are infrequently isolated from swine and are of questionable pathogenicity. These include *M. arginini, M. bovigenitalium, M. buccale, M. hyopharyngis, M. gallinarum, M. iners, M. mycoides* subsp. *mycoides, M. salivarium, M. sualvi, Acholeplasma axanthum, A. granularum, A. laidlawii* and *A. oculi.*[16,25] *Ureaplasma* has been isolated from swine semen by a group of Hungarian researchers.[22] Efforts by others to recover ureaplasmas from the porcine reproductive tract have been unsuccessful.

Mycoplasma hyopneumoniae

Mycoplasma hyopneumoniae is the causative agent of mycoplasmal pneumonia of swine (MPS), or enzootic pneumonia of pigs.[12,13,16,25] This disease occurs in all of the swine-rearing regions of the world. It has a high attack rate; essentially every conventional herd is affected. Morbidity is high, but mortality is near zero. The disease is characterized by a chronic nonproductive cough, retarded growth rate, and inefficient utilization of

---

*Editor's note: Since Metricel GA-8 filter media (see p. 72) are no longer available, Durapore GVWP filter media (Millipore Corporation, Bedford, MA) can be substituted. These filters will clear in IF buffer with 50% glycerol.

feed. It is an economically important disease due to the poor growth and poor feed utilization. Annual losses in the United States have been estimated to be $200 million[24] and $330 million.[7]

Gross lesions occur most frequently in the anterior lobes of the lungs. They are lobular in distribution and purple to gray in color. In the acute phase of the disease the lobules are swollen and the airways contain copious amounts of a sticky white exudate. Such lungs are ideal diagnostic specimens since the causative agent is present in large numbers. Chronic phase lesions are contracted rather than swollen and contain the causative agent in low numbers. Gross lung lesions seen in market swine reflect a mixed mycoplasmal and bacterial pneumonia and may not fit the description given above.

Most laboratories diagnose MPS solely on the basis of lung lesions, but while these are characteristic, they are not pathognomonic. Furthermore, *M. hyopneumoniae* is frequently present in lungs that are grossly normal. Thus, sole reliance on lesions can lead to both false positive and false negative diagnoses.[4] A definitive diagnosis of MPS requires that *M. hyopneumoniae* be visualized in immunofluorescent (IF)-stained lung sections or that the agent be recovered culturally. Though IF staining is a simple, inexpensive and practical method of diagnosing MPS, false negative results do occur. Therefore, the following approach is recommended: (1) lung specimens are collected for both cultural and IF studies; (2) the specimens for cultural examination are stored in the refrigerator or freezer until IF studies are complete; and (3) the tissues collected for IF studies are stained and examined microscopically for the presence of *M. hyopneumoniae*. Positive IF results are reliable (provided, of course, that reagents are specific, that adequate controls are used and that the technician is properly trained). Therefore, if *M. hyopneumoniae* is detected in the IF-stained sections, a diagnosis of MPS can be made, and the specimen stored for cultural examination can be discarded without further study. When the IF examination is negative, the stored specimen should be examined culturally for mycoplasmas.

Harvesting Tissues for Immunofluorescent and Cultural Studies

The preferred specimen for the laboratory diagnosis of MPS is a lung from a pig in the acute phase of the disease. In chronically affected herds (which means most of the herds of the world) a significant percentage of swine will have typical acute phase lesions at about 4 months of age. Lungs from such swine will be heavily colonized with *M. hyopneumoniae*. A high percentage of market swine will have gross lesions of pneumonia. However, many of the lungs from such swine will be culturally negative for *M. hyo-*

pneumoniae (although culturally positive for bacteria such as *Pasteurella multocida* and *Streptococcus suis*).

It is recommended that a portion of each of the four anterior lobes be examined because it is these lobes that usually harbor the greatest number of *M. hyopneumoniae* organisms. Specimens are collected from the advancing (dorsal) margin of the lesion so as to include both diseased and normal tissue. In the absence of lesions, specimens are collected from the ventral margin of the lobe. Surface contaminants must be removed from the specimens that are harvested for cultural examination. Therefore, they are collected first and then adjacent specimens are collected for IF studies.

Small lungs are decontaminated as follows. The lobe to be examined is clamped at the hilus with a pair of large surgical forceps and severed, transversely, proximal to the forceps. The lobe, held by the forceps, is immersed in boiling water for eight seconds, and the excess water is shaken off. The lobe is held over a sterile beaker or regular-size Tekmar Lab Bag (Tekmar, Cincinnati, OH) containing 10 ml of grinding medium (see Appendix A6.1 at the end of this chapter). A portion of tissue about 1 cm³ is snipped off and allowed to fall into the medium. The procedure is repeated with the remaining three lobes. With larger lungs, the areas to be sampled are seared to a depth of about ¹⁄₁₆th of an inch with a hot spatula or a propane torch. Blocks of tissue, about 1 cm³, are then removed aseptically with sterile scissors and forceps and transferred to a sterile beaker or plastic bag containing 10 ml of grinding medium.

The specimens collected from the four anterior lobes and placed in grinding medium are macerated in a mortar and pestle or in a Stomacher Lab Blender 80 (Fisher Scientific, Springfield, NJ). A portion of the tissue suspension is inoculated onto bacteriologic culture medium and the remainder is stored in a refrigerator or freezer until IF studies are complete. The bacteriologic media are incubated appropriately and significant bacterial colonies that develop are subsequently identified.

Immunofluorescent Examination of Lungs

A block of tissue about 1 cm³ is collected adjacent to each of the specimens harvested for cultural studies. Each block is mounted on a cryostat object holder in Tissue-Tek O.C.T. Compound (American Scientific Products, McGaw Park, IL) so that airways will be cut transversely. It is frozen, and two sections are cut and mounted side by side on a microscope slide. The sections are air dried and fixed in acetone for 10 minutes. A heavy line is drawn between the two tissue sections with a warm wax pencil. One of the tissue sections is reacted with antiserum to *M. hyopneumoniae* and the other is reacted with normal serum. Either the direct or indirect method of immunofluorescent staining may be used (see Chapter 3). The author prefers the indirect method using antiserum prepared in rabbits and commercially prepared anti-rabbit serum conjugated with fluorescein isothiocyanate. A slide with two sections from a lung known to be infected with *M. hyopneumoniae* is stained the same way, as positive and negative controls. The slides are examined with a fluorescence microscope. The control slide is examined first. The section reacted with *M. hyopneumoniae* antiserum should be clearly positive; i.e., brightly staining particles and aggregates of *M. hyopneumoniae* should be present on the surface of the bronchial and bronchiolar epithelium (Fig. 6.1). The negative control section should be clearly negative; i.e., it should be devoid of fluorescing elements. Once the microscopist is assured that the controls are satisfactory, the diagnostic specimens are examined. The section reacted with the *M. hyopneumoniae* antiserum is examined first. If it is negative there is no need to examine the section reacted with the normal serum. If, however, it is positive the section reacted with the normal serum should be examined to be sure the fluorescence is not an artifact. Fluorescing elements seen anywhere other than the surface of the bronchial and bronchiolar epithelium should be regarded as artifacts.

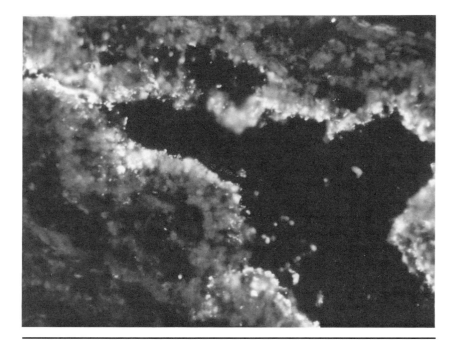

Fig. 6.1. *Mycoplasma hyopneumoniae*-infected lung stained by the indirect immunofluorescent method. The brightly stained particles on the surface of the bronchial epithelium are individual mycoplasmal cells and aggregates of cells.

Cultural Examination

The tissue suspension, prepared as described above, is used as inoculum. It is removed from storage, thawed if frozen, and 0.5 ml is inoculated into 4.5 ml of Friis' broth[11] supplemented with cycloserine and *M. hyorhinis* antiserum (see appendix at the end of this chapter). This first dilution is identified as a 10^{-2} dilution (the tissue suspended in grinding medium is assumed to be a 10^{-1} dilution). Two additional 10-fold serial dilutions are prepared (0.5 ml of inoculum and 4.5 ml of Friis' broth) and identified as 10^{-3} and 10^{-4} dilutions. The inoculated broths are incubated at 37°C in a roller drum turned at approximately 0.5 rpm. *M. hyopneumoniae* grows better when turned in a roller drum, so this step should not be neglected when attempting to isolate the organism from lung tissue.[11]

Inoculated broths are examined daily for (1) turbidity and (2) pH change. Bacterial contamination occurs in the lower dilutions fairly often despite decontamination efforts and the incorporation of antibiotics in the culture broth. Bacterial growth is characterized by heavy turbidity and, usually, a pH shift. Growth of *M. hyopneumoniae,* on the other hand, is characterized by little, if any, turbidity and an acid shift in pH (the broth turns from the original salmon color to a yellow color). *M. hyopneumoniae* grows fairly slowly; in heavily infected lungs the first pH change occurs about 5 or 6 days postincubation. A pH change may not be seen for 14 days or more when the lung contains only small numbers of *M. hyopneumoniae* organisms. There are two other respiratory mycoplasmas of swine that also induce an acid pH change in Friis' broth, viz., *M. flocculare* and *M. hyorhinis. M. flocculare* is a fastidious mycoplasma that grows at about the same rate as *M. hyopneumoniae. M. hyorhinis,* a very common inhabitant of the porcine respiratory tract, grows rapidly and may appear 2 or 3 days postincubation. However, the incorporation of cycloserine and *M. hyorhinis* antiserum into Friis' broth effectively suppresses the growth of *M. hyorhinis.* It is very important to incorporate these reagents into Friis' broth when attempting to isolate *M. hyopneumoniae;* otherwise, *M. hyorhinis* is apt to overgrow the culture.

Identification procedures are initiated as soon as a culture becomes acid, assuming an absence of the turbidity that occurs with bacterial growth. *M. hyopneumoniae* is reluctant to colonize agar when first isolated from tissue. Therefore, the usual methods of identification (i.e., growth inhibition and IF staining of colonies on agar) cannot be used unless the isolate is first subcultured in broth for two or three passages. To overcome this difficulty, (1) aseptically pass 2 ml of a 10^{-1} dilution of the primary culture through a sterile 0.20 μm, 47 mm filter membrane (Metricel GA-8, Gelman Instrument Co., Ann Arbor, MI)* in a 47 mm funnel and base (Analytical Filter Holder, Millipore Corporation, Bedford, MA). (2) Immerse the inoculated membrane in Friis' broth and (3) incubate the preparation in a candle jar at 37°C for 5 or 6 days. (4) Remove and wash the membrane in buffer, and (5) stain small segments of the membrane by the indirect IF procedure.[1] Direct IF staining probably could also be used. Passing a primary culture through a filter membrane and subsequent incubation of the preparation in culture broth results in the formation of colonies on the membrane surface. (The appearance of *M. hyopneumoniae* colonies grown on a filter membrane and stained by the indirect IF procedure is illustrated in Figure 6.2.) This technique can be used to identify any species of mycoplasma. The membranes are easier to handle than agar blocks (see Chapter 3) and there is almost no background fluorescence, provided a filter membrane is used that does not absorb proteins. It has been learned recently that the incubation step can be eliminated. The procedure currently used in the author's laboratory is to pass 2 ml of a 10^{-1} dilution of a primary culture through a non-sterile 25 mm 0.20 μm filter (Metricel GA-8, Gelman) in a 25 mm plastic Swinney holder (Swinnex, Millipore Corporation, Bedford, MA). The membrane is removed from the holder, labeled, washed in buffer, cut into sections and stained. Details of this procedure are illustrated in Figure 6.3. Colonies are not formed when

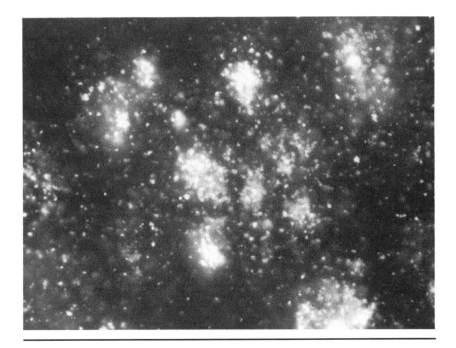

Fig. 6.2. Colonies of *Mycoplasma hyopneumoniae* grown on a filter membrane and stained by the indirect immunofluorescent method. The loose nebulous nature of the colonies is typical of *Mycoplasma hyopneumoniae*.

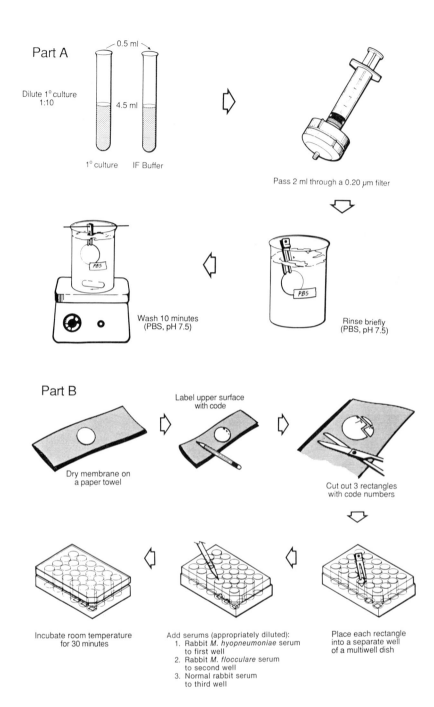

Part A

Dilute 1° culture 1:10

0.5 ml

4.5 ml

1° culture   IF Buffer

Pass 2 ml through a 0.20 μm filter

Wash 10 minutes (PBS, pH 7.5)

Rinse briefly (PBS, pH 7.5)

Part B

Dry membrane on a paper towel

Label upper surface with code

Cut out 3 rectangles with code numbers

Incubate room temperature for 30 minutes

Add serums (appropriately diluted):
1. Rabbit *M. hyopneumoniae* serum to first well
2. Rabbit *M. flocculare* serum to second well
3. Normal rabbit serum to third well

Place each rectangle into a separate well of a multiwell dish

Fig. 6.3. Details of the membrane technique of identifying mycoplasmas. A. Collection of organisms and initial cleansing. B. Drying, labeling, adding primary antisera, and incubating. C. Second cleansing, drying, adding "conjugate," incubating, third cleansing, and drying. D. Preparation and observation of slides.

74

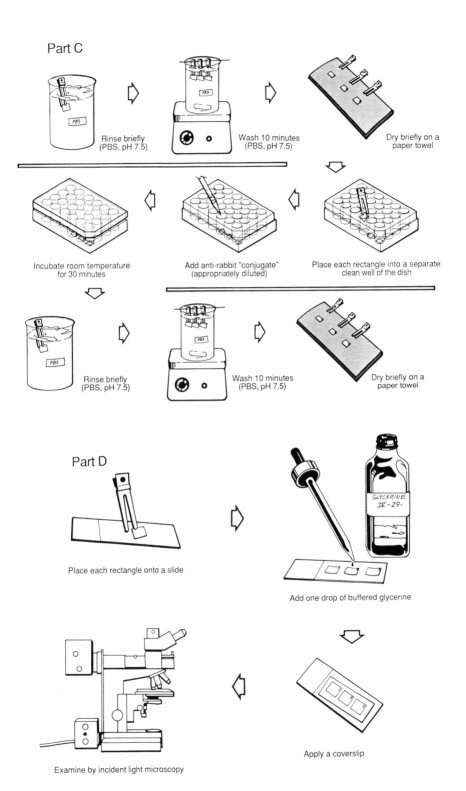

Part C

Rinse briefly
(PBS, pH 7.5)

Wash 10 minutes
(PBS, pH 7.5)

Dry briefly on a
paper towel

Incubate room temperature
for 30 minutes

Add anti-rabbit "conjugate"
(appropriately diluted)

Place each rectangle into a separate
clean well of the dish

Rinse briefly
(PBS, pH 7.5)

Wash 10 minutes
(PBS, pH 7.5)

Dry briefly on a
paper towel

Part D

Place each rectangle onto a slide

Add one drop of buffered glycerine

Apply a coverslip

Examine by incident light microscopy

75

the incubation step is eliminated. However, *M. hyopneumoniae* forms modest to large aggregates when first isolated from tissue, and these aggregates adhere to the membrane and stain brightly with appropriate IF reagents. (It should be noted that *M. flocculare* forms *very* large aggregates when first recovered from tissue, so the difference in the size of the aggregates of the two species is an additional aid in identification.)

There are a few details of identifying mycoplasmas by IF staining of organisms on membranes that need to be emphasized. Some filter membranes absorb serum proteins non-specifically, which causes a high level of background staining. The filter recommended herein does not have this undesirable characteristic. It is important to maintain orientation so that the stained section is mounted surface-side-up. One way to do this is to apply a numerical code on the upper right corner of the membrane section. This code also is used to identify the antiserum applied to the section. The indirect IF procedure is recommended. Three sections are routinely stained, i.e., one each is reacted with antiserum to *M. hyopneumoniae* and *M. flocculare* and one with normal serum. Stained sections are examined with an incident light microscope, i.e., by epifluorescence. Antisera to both *M. hyopneumoniae* and *M. flocculare* are used in order to detect mixed cultures. This approach also serves as a quality control for evaluating the primary antisera. *M. hyopneumoniae* and *M. flocculare* share common antigens, and hyperimmune antiserum to each of these species cross-react with the other. Consequently, the primary antiserum should be absorbed with whole cells of the heterologous species. Absorption is accomplished as follows: 10 ml of *M. hyopneumoniae* antiserum is mixed with cells collected by centrifugation from 100 ml of *M. flocculare* culture. The suspension is incubated for 1 hour at 37°C and overnight at 4°C. The antiserum is then recovered by centrifugation. Antiserum to *M. flocculare* is absorbed with whole cells of *M. hyopneumoniae* in the same way. Controls consist of membranes inoculated with type cultures of *M. hyopneumoniae* and *M. flocculare* reacted with homologous and heterologous antisera and normal serum.

Serology

Serodiagnosis of MPS is sometimes useful on a herd basis, but may not rule in or rule out the disease in an individual animal, as currently available tests lack sensitivity and/or specificity.[2] The test most readily available in the United States is the complement fixation (CF) test.[21] The CF test is useful in detecting early infection, but individual swine may become CF negative in the later stages of infection (Armstrong CH, Freeman MJ, et al.: 1982, Unpublished data). The enzyme-linked immunosorbent assay (ELISA) has the advantage of being very sensitive.[2,6] However, like all serologic tests currently available, the ELISA lacks specificity. Non-specific reactions are due to the crude antigens employed (whole-cell or membrane lysates). Antigens extracted with polysorbate reportedly are more specific than those prepared with sodium dodecyl sulphate.[15]

Mycoplasma hyorhinis

Mycoplasma hyorhinis is a common inhabitant of the upper respiratory tract of swine.[20,24] It occasionally causes polyarthritis and polyserositis in swine, usually during the first 10 weeks of life.[16]

A definitive diagnosis of *M. hyorhinis*–induced disease requires that the causative agent be isolated and identified. It must particularly be distinguished from Glasser's disease. *M. hyorhinis* is a rapid growing organism and, like *M. hyopneumoniae,* it causes an acid shift in culture broth.

Cultural Examination and Serology

Specimens selected for cultural studies vary according to the manifestation(s) of the disease. Joint fluid and/or synovial membrane are examined in cases of polyarthritis. Pleura, pericardium and/or peritoneum are examined in the polyserositis cases. Most strains of *M. hyorhinis* will grow in a variety of mycoplasma culture media. Friis' broth, without cycloserine and anti-*hyorhinis* serum, is used in the author's laboratory. Three or four 10-fold dilutions are prepared (0.5 ml of inoculum and 4.5 ml of Friis' broth). Synovial and serous membranes are macerated in grinding medium (as described above for isolation of *M. hyopneumoniae*) and then diluted in culture broth. Joint fluid is diluted in culture broth without prior treatment. The inoculated media are incubated at 37°C and examined daily for turbidity and pH change. As described above, bacterial contamination, which may occur in the lower dilution(s), is characterized by turbidity and, usually, an acid or alkaline pH change. Growth of *M. hyorhinis* is characterized by an acid pH change and only slight turbidity. Identification procedures are initiated when a broth becomes acid without extreme turbidity. It is recommended that *M. hyorhinis* suspects be identified by IF staining of colonies grown on filter membranes or on agar (Friis' broth solidified with 1% Noble agar). The growth inhibition test (described in Chapter 3) can be used, but results may not be definitive due to the antigenic diversity that occurs among different strains of *M. hyorhinis.*[25]

There is no serological test available for general diagnostic use.

Mycoplasma hyosynoviae

Mycoplasma hyosynoviae is a fairly rapid growing mycoplasma that hydrolyzes arginine.[18] It is a common inhabitant of the upper respiratory tract that occasionally causes polyarthritis, usually in swine that are 12–24 weeks of age.[16] A definitive diagnosis of *M. hyosynoviae* arthritis requires that the organism be recovered from affected joints.

Cultural Examination and Serology

The cultural examination should be performed during the acute phase of the disease because *M. hyosynoviae* disappears from affected joints after about 3 weeks.[19] Either joint fluid or synovial membrane may be examined. Synovial membrane is first macerated in grinding medium (10^{-1} dilution). Three or four serial 10-fold dilutions are then prepared in hyosynoviae (HS) broth (see appendix at the end of this chapter): 0.5 ml of inoculum and 4.5 ml of HS. Cultures are incubated at 37°C and examined daily. As described previously, bacterial contamination may occur in the lower dilution(s), and is characterized by turbidity and usually a pH shift. Growth of *M. hyosynoviae* is characterized by lack of heavy turbidity, an alkaline pH shift (the broth changes from the initial salmon color to a deep reddish blue) and the formation of a pellicle. Soap-like deposits usually form on the wall of the test tube. When the latter features are observed, identification procedures are initiated. *Mycoplasma hyosynoviae* can be identified by any of the methods previously described: the growth inhibition test or by IF staining of colonies grown on agar, or by IF staining of organisms on a filter membrane. The medium used to grow colonies on agar is HS broth solidified with 1% Noble agar. Most strains of *M. hyosynoviae* will form films and spots on this agar. This change is seen as a pearlescent "crystalline" deposit over the mycoplasma colonies.

There is no serologic test available for diagnosing *M. hyosynoviae* infections.

In conclusion, three species of mycoplasmas commonly cause diseases in swine: *M. hyopneumoniae, M. hyorhinis* and *M. hyosynoviae.*

Mycoplasma hyopneumoniae, the causative agent of MPS, is the most important economically. It is diagnosed by visualizing the agent in infected airways or by recovering the organism culturally from infected lungs. Visualization requires that the agent be stained with a specific immunological reagent. Immunofluorescence is commonly used and requires a fluorescence microscope. There are other immunostaining procedures that allow the antigen to be visualized with a regular bright light microscope, e.g., peroxidase-antiperoxidase and biotin-avidin-peroxidase[5] (which are very sensitive but not currently in use for diagnosing MPS). Sole reliance on lung lesions can result in both false negative and false positive diagnoses. Serology is not reliable for identifying individually infected swine. *Mycoplasma hyorhinis* causes polyarthritis/polyserositis in young swine. Infections generally are sporadic and characterized by low morbidity. Disease caused by *M. hyorhinis* must be differentiated from Glasser's disease. A diagnosis of *M. hyorhinis* infection requires that the organism be recovered from diseased tissues. There is no serologic test available to the diagnostician.

Mycoplasma hyosynoviae causes polyarthritis in older swine. It, too, is generally a sporadic infection characterized by low morbidity. This disease is diagnosed by isolating the causative agent from affected joints. No serologic test is available.

References

1. Armstrong CH: 1977, A diagnostically practical method of isolating and identifying *Mycoplasma hyopneumoniae*. Proc I Simposium Internacional De Laboratorios de Diagnostico, Guanajuato, Mexico, 754–771.

2. Armstrong CH, Freeman MJ, Sands Freeman L, Lopez Osuna M, Young T, Runnels LJ: 1983, Comparison of the enzyme-linked immunosorbent assay and the indirect hemagglutination and complement fixation tests for detecting antibodies to *Mycoplasma hyopneumoniae*. Can J Comp Med 47:464–470.

3. Armstrong CH, Friis NF: 1981, Isolation of *Mycoplasma flocculare* from swine in the United States. Am J Vet Res 42:1030–1032.

4. Armstrong CH, Scheidt AB, Thacker HL, Runnels LJ, Freeman MJ: 1984, Evaluation of criteria for the postmortem diagnosis of mycoplasmal pneumonia of swine. Can J Comp Med 48:278–281.

5. Bourne JA: 1983, Handbook of Immunoperoxidase Staining Methods. Immunochemistry Laboratory, Dako Corporation, Santa Barbara, CA 93103.

6. Bruggmann S, Keller H, Bertschinger HU, Ingbert B: 1977, Quantitative detection of antibodies to *Mycoplasma suipneumoniae* in pigs' sera by an enzyme-linked immunosorbent assay. Vet Rec 101:109–111.

7. Clark LK: 1987, School of Vet Med, Purdue University, West Lafayette, IN. Personal communication.

8. Friis NF: 1972, Isolation and characterization of a new porcine mycoplasma. Acta Vet Scand 13:284–286.

9. Friis NF: 1973, The pathogenicity of *Mycoplasma flocculare*. Acta Vet Scand 14:344–346.

10. Friis NF: 1974, *Mycoplasma suipneumoniae* and *Mycoplasma flocculare* in comparative pathogenicity studies. Acta Vet Scand 15:507–518.

11. Friis NF: 1975, Some recommendations concerning primary isolation of *Mycoplasma suipneumoniae* and *Mycoplasma flocculare*. Nord Vet Med 27:337–339.

12. Goodwin RFW, Pomeroy AP, Whittlestone P: 1965, Production of enzootic pneumonia in pigs with a mycoplasma. Vet Rec 77:1247–1249.

13. Mare CJ, Switzer WP: 1965, New species; *Mycoplasma hyopneumoniae,* a causative agent of virus pig pneumonia. Vet Med 60:841–846.

14. Meyling A, Friis NF: 1972, Serological identification of a new porcine mycoplasma species, *M. flocculare.* Acta Vet Scand 13:287–289.

15. Nicolet J, Paroz P, Bruggmann S: 1980, Tween 20 soluble proteins of *Mycoplasma hyopneumoniae* as antigen for an enzyme-linked immunosorbent assay. Res Vet Sci 29:305–309.

16. Ross RF: 1986, Mycoplasmal diseases. In: Diseases of Swine, ed. Leman AD, Straw BE, Glock RD, Mengeling WL, Penny RHC, Scholl E, 6th ed., pp. 469–483. Iowa State University Press, Ames, IA.

17. Ross RF, Karmon JA: 1970, Heterogeneity among strains of *Mycoplasma granularum* and identification of *Mycoplasma hyosynoviae,* sp. n. J Bacteriol 103:707–713.

18. Ross RF, Spear ML: 1973, Role of the sow as a reservoir of infection for *Mycoplasma hyosynoviae.* Am J Vet Res 34:373–378.

19. Ross RF, Switzer WP, Duncan JR: 1971, Experimental production of *Mycoplasma hyosynoviae* arthritis in swine. Am J Vet Res 32:1743–1749.

20. Schulman A, Estola T, Garry-Andersson AS: 1970, On the occurrence of *Mycoplasma hyorhinis* in the respiratory organs of pigs, with special reference to enzootic pneumonia. Zentralbl Veterinaermed 17:549–553.

21. Slavik MF, Switzer WP: 1972, Development of a microtitration complement-fixation test for diagnosis of mycoplasmal swine pneumonia. Iowa State J Res 47:117–128.

22. Stipkovits L, Rashwan A, Takacs J, Lapis K: 1978, Occurrence of ureaplasmas in swine semen. Zentralbl Veterinaermed (B) 25:605–608.

23. Switzer WP: 1955, Studies on infectious atrophic rhinitis. IV. Characterization of a pleuropneumonia-like organism isolated from the nasal cavities of swine. Am J Vet Res 16:540–544.

24. Switzer WP, Ross RF: 1975, Mycoplasmal diseases, In: Diseases of Swine, eds. Dunne HW, Leman AD, 4th ed., pp. 741–764. Iowa State University Press, Ames, IA.

25. Whittlestone P: 1979, Porcine mycoplasmas. In: The Mycoplasmas, eds. Tully JG, Whitcomb RF, pp. 133–176. Academic Press, New York, NY.

Appendix A6.1

Grinding Medium

HBSS-Part A	40.0 ml
HBSS-Part B	40.0 ml
Brain Heart Infusion Broth	
(Difco Laboratories, Detroit, MI)	5.0 g
PPLO Broth w/o crystal violet (Difco)	5.2 g
Deionized water (cell culture quality)	1170.0 ml

Dissolve and sterilize at 15 psi/3 minutes in a pressure cooker containing deionized water. (An autoclave with a central steam supply is not recommended due to the possibility of toxic products being present in the steam.) Cool and dispense in 100-ml aliquots, e.g., in sterile plastic cups with sterile lids (Falcon Division, Becton Dickinson & Co., Oxnard, CA). Label and store at −40°F.

Friis' Broth

HBSS-Part A	40.0 ml
HBSS-Part B	40.0 ml
Brain Heart Infusion Broth	
(Difco Laboratories, Detroit, MI)	5.0 g
PPLO Broth w/o crystal violet (Difco)	5.2 g
Deionized water (cell culture quality)	1170.0 ml

Dissolve, sterilize at 15 psi/3 minutes in a pressure cooker containing deionized water, cool, and add the following sterilized ingredients:

Yeast extract	60.0 ml
Bacitracin (5000 units/ml)	2.9 ml
Methicillin (100 mg/ml)	2.5 ml
Phenol red (0.5% solution)	4.5 ml
Swine serum (56° C/30 min)	165.0 ml
Horse serum	165.0 ml

Adjust pH to 7.5 or 7.6. Dispense in 100-ml amounts in sterile plastic cups with sterile lids (Falcon Division, Becton Dickinson & Co., Oxnard, CA). Label and store at −40°F.

For isolation of *M. hyopneumoniae* from lungs of conventional swine, add *M. hyorhinis* antiserum (5 ml/100 ml of Friis' broth) and cycloserine (0.5 mg/ml of Friis' broth).

Hyosynoviae (HS) Broth

PPLO Broth w/o crystal violet (Difco)	10.3 g
Deionized water	470.0 ml

Sterilize at 15 psi/3 minutes in a pressure cooker containing deionized water, cool, and add the following sterilized ingredients:

Yeast extract	25.0 ml
Penicillin G (100,000 units/ml)	1.5 ml
Thallium acetate (5.6% solution)	1.2 ml
Phenol red solution (0.5% solution)	1.8 ml
Arginine-mucin suspension	16.0 ml
Turkey serum (56°C/30 min)	129.0 ml

Adjust pH to 7.2; dispense in 100-ml amounts in sterile cups with sterile lids, label, and store at −40°F.

Modified Hanks' Balanced Salt Solution (HBSS)
Part A

NaCl	80 g
KCl	4 g
$MgSO_4 \cdot 7H_2O$	1 g
$MgCl_2 \cdot 6H_2O$	1 g

Dissolve in 400 ml of deionized water. Add 1.4 g $CaCl_2$ and QS to 500 ml with deionized water. Label and store at 4°C.

Part B
Dissolve 1.5 g $Na_2HPO_4 \cdot 12H_2O$ in 400 ml deionized water. Add 0.6 g KH_2PO_4 and QS to 500 ml with deionized water. Label and store at 4°C.

Yeast Extract for Friis' Broth
Suspend 125 g dry *Saccharomyces cerevesiae* (Red Star Active Dry Yeast, Universal Foods corporation, Milwaukee, WI) in 750 ml deionized water and place in 37°C water bath 20 minutes. Place in a boiling water bath 5 minutes, cool, centrifuge, remove supernatant fluid and filter through a Whatman #1 (Whatman Inc., Paper Division, Clifton, NJ). Sterilize at 15psi/3 minutes in a pressure cooker containing deionized water, cool, dispense in sterile cups with sterile lids in 60 ml amounts, label and store at −40°F.

Note: There may be a precipitate when the extract is removed from the pressure cooker; this precipitate will dissolve when the extract cools.

Yeast Extract for HS Broth
Suspend 250 g dry yeast in 1 liter deionized water. Follow instructions for preparing yeast extract for Friis' broth. Dispense sterilized extract in 25-ml amounts, label, and store at −40°F.

Bacitracin Solution
Dissolve 50,000 units of Bacitracin (The Upjohn Company, Kalamazoo, MI) in 10 ml deionized water. Pass through a sterile disposable 0.22 μm Swinney filter (Millex, Millipore Corporation, Bedford, MA). Dispense in 2.9-ml amounts, label and store at −40°F.

Methicillin Solution
Dissolve 1 g of methicillin (Staphcillin, methicillin sodium for injection, Bristol Laboratories, Inc., Evansville, IN) in 10 ml of deionized water. Pass through a sterile disposable 0.22 μm Swinney filter, dispense in 2.5-ml amounts, label and store at −40°F.

Phenol Red Solution
Grind 2.5 g of phenol red in a mortar with successive additions of 0.1N NaOH until 75 ml has been added. Bring to 500 ml with deionized water and refrigerate (4°C) overnight. Filter through a #1 Whatman filter, adjust pH to 7.0, dispense in 4.5- and 1.8-ml aliquots and sterilize at 15psi/3 minutes in a pressure cooker containing deionized water. Cool, label, and store at −40°F.

Penicillin G Solution
Dissolve 1,000,000 units of crystalline penicillin G in 10 ml of deionized water. Pass through a sterile disposable 0.22 μm Swinney filter, dispense in 1.5-ml amounts, label, and store at −40°F.

Thallium Acetate Solution
Dissolve 1.12 g of thallium acetate in 20 ml of deionized water. Pass through a sterile disposable 0.22 μm Swinney filter, dispense in 1.2-ml amounts, label and store at −40°.

Arginine-Mucin Suspension
Dissolve 8 g of arginine monochloride in 100 ml of deionized water and suspend 0.8 g of Bacto mucin (Difco) in the solution. Sterilize at 15 psi/3 minutes in a pressure cooker containing deionized water, aseptically dispense (keeping suspension well mixed) in 16-ml amounts, label, and store at −40°F.

Buffer for Immunofluorescent (IF) Staining

$NaH_2PO_4 \cdot H_2O$	24	g
$NaH_2PO_4 \cdot HOH$	4.4	g
NaCl	170	g
Deionized water	2000	ml

Add compounds one at a time to the water. When all are in solution add 4 g NaN_3. Dilute an aliquot 1:10 and test pH, which should be 7.3–7.6. If pH is correct, pour into a 5-gallon carboy and add 18,000 ml of deionized water. Label "Working IF Buffer" and store at room temperature.

CHAPTER 7

Ovine and Caprine Mycoplasmas

S. ROSENDAL

With few exceptions, sheep and goats share their mycoplasma flora. This can undoubtedly be explained by the close phylogenetic relationship of these two animal species, although host adaptation needs to be studied at the cellular and molecular levels. Table 7.1 lists the mycoplasmas isolated from sheep and goats and disease associations, preferred culture media, and serodiagnostic methods reported for each species.* If isolates from sheep or goats cannot be identified as one of the species or taxa listed in Table 7.1, the routine diagnostic laboratory should look next to the bovine mycoplasma flora. When isolates of uncertain identity are encountered, it is important that these be placed in reference laboratories for more complete taxonomical studies.

―――――
Gratitude is expressed to Dr. G.E. Jones, Animal Diseases Research Association, Moredun Research Institute, Edinburgh for comments and suggestions to improve the manuscript.
*Readers are referred to a comprehensive review published while this book was in press: DaMassa AJ, Wakenell PS, Brooks DL: 1992, Mycoplasmas of goats and sheep. J Vet Diagn Invest 4: 101–113. In addition, gene probes and polymerase-chain-reaction-based diagnostic techniques have been reported for some bovine and caprine mycoplasmas: Dedieu SCL, Breard A, Bensaid A, Lefevre P-C: 1992, Development of species-specific DNA probes for *Mycoplasma capricolum, Mycoplasma agalactiae* and *Mycoplasma mycoides* subsp. *mycoides* SC. IOM Letters 2: 203; and Taylor TK, Bashiruddin J, Gould AR: 1992, Development of a test based on the Polymerase Chain Reaction (PCR) for the specific identification of *Mycoplasma mycoides* subsp. *mycoides* SC. IOM Letters 2: 107.

Table 7.1. Overview of ovine-caprine mycoplasmas, disease association, habitat, preferred culture medium, and serodiagnostic methods

Agent	Disease Association or Habitat	Culture Medium	Serodiagnostic Method
M. agalactiae	Contagious agalactia syndrome (S + G)[a]	H[b]	ELISA, CF
M. mycoides subsp. mycoides LC-type	Septicemia, arthritis, pleuropneumonia, mastitis, conjunctivitis (G)	H	CF, IHA
M. mycoides subsp. capri	Pleuropneumonia, septicemia, arthritis, mastitis (G)	H	CF, IHA
M. capricolum	Pleuropneumonia, septicemia, arthritis, mastitis, abscesses, conjunctivitis (S + G)	H	CF, IHA
Taxon F-38	Contagious caprine pleuropneumoniae	WJ[c]	CF, IHA
M. ovipneumoniae	Pneumonia, pleuritis (S + G)	F[d]	IHA, ELISA
M. arginini	Respiratory and genital tract (S + G)	H	IHA
M. putrefaciens	Mastitis, arthritis (G)	H	CF, TA
M. conjunctivae	Keratoconjunctivitis (S + G)	H	MIT, ELISA
Taxon 2D	Vulvovaginitis (S)	H	–[f]
Taxon G, U, V	Ear	H	–
Ureaplasmas	Urogenital and respiratory tract (S + G)	U[e]	–
A. oculi	Keratoconjunctivitis (S + G)	H	–
A. laidlawii	All mucosal membranes	H	–

[a]Bracketed letters indicate host species (sheep/goat)
[b]H: medium based on Hayflick's formula
[c]Wood and Jones' formula
[d]Friis' formula
[e]Ureaplasma medium
[f]No method described

Mycoplasma agalactiae

This mycoplasma causes contagious agalactia of sheep and goats, one of the most important mycoplasma diseases.[13] Serious outbreaks may involve close to 100% of the susceptible animals, of which 10–20% may die. The disease occurs in most Mediterranean countries and in Africa and Asia. *M. agalactiae* has been isolated in both Australia and the United States, but the typical contagious disease is apparently not present. The infection spreads by carriers, and outbreaks with high morbidity may occur when they are introduced into a herd of susceptible animals. Unilateral or bilateral acute mastitis leading to virtually complete agalactia results from infection of the mammary gland. The mastitis may progress to septicemia and death in some of the affected animals, and secondary arthritis and keratoconjunctivitis are common sequelae in surviving animals. Genital tract infections have been reported from India.[28]

Mammary secretions, joint taps, and eye and ear swabs are suitable for culture. Herd screening may be achieved by culturing bulk milk samples. The likelihood of isolating the organism from blood is relatively low even if several samples are taken during the acute phase. *M. agalactiae* grows well on media based on Hayflick's formula (see Appendix A7.1 at the end of this chapter). The number of mycoplasmas in mastitis secretions may fluctuate considerably, making it necessary to culture several samples taken on different days. The direct staining of secretions with acridine orange may be useful for differentiating mycoplasma infections from bacterial infections.[11] The biochemical reactions of *M. agalactiae* are listed in Table 7.2. The failure to ferment glucose and hydrolyse arginine is highly suggestive of *M. agalactiae,* but needs to be confirmed by serological identification using the growth inhibition (GI) or fluorescent antibody (FA) test. Antibodies detected by ELISA[27], complement fixation (CF), or a test based on inhibition of the "Film and Spots" reaction are evidence of exposure to *M. agalactiae* infection.

M. mycoides subspecies *mycoides,* Large Colony–Type (LC-type)

During the past decade, diseases of goats caused by a mycoplasma with important antigens in common with *M. mycoides* subsp. *mycoides* have been recognized in many countries free of contagious bovine pleuropneumonia (CBPP), such as the United States and Canada. The bovine variant can be distinguished from the caprine variant by several features, of which colony size is the most practical. The bovine variant differs from the caprine variant in producing relatively small colonies ≤0.5 mm (≥1 mm for caprine variants), being non-caseinolytic, sensitive to heat at 45°C, and failing to grow on 5% sheep blood agar. Veterinary diagnostic laboratories may isolate this organism on routine sheep or calf blood agar and mistake it for a fastidious α-hemolytic *Streptococcus* until the failure to recognize bacteria in a Gram-stained smear prompts subculture onto a mycoplasma medium.[26]

The LC-type causes septicemia and polyarthritis in young goats, and occasionally pneumonia.[23] Older animals may suffer from mastitis and shed large numbers in the milk, which in turn may cause septicemia if fed unpasteurized to kids.[7] Adult goats may also develop arthritis, keratoconjunctivitis, and outer ear infection as a result of mycoplasmaemia or self-inoculation of the eye and ear.

The LC-type is often isolated from lungs and pleural exudate of goats with diseases mimicking contagious caprine pleuropneumonia (CCPP). If isolated from classical CCPP it would play a secondary role to the F-38

Table 7.2. Useful biochemical reactions for initial screening of ovine and caprine mycoplasma isolates

	Digitonin Sensitivity	Urease Activity	Glucose Fermentation	Arginine hydrolysis	Phosphatase Activity	"Film & Spots"	Caseinolytic Activity
M. agalactiae	+	−	−	−	+	+	−
M. mycoides subsp. mycoides LC-type	+	−	+	−	−	−	+
M. mycoides subsp. mycoides SC-type	+	−	+	−	−	−	+
M. mycoides subsp. capri	+	−	+	−	−	−	+
M. capricolum	+	−	+	(+)[a]	+	−	+
Taxon F-38	+	−	+	−	−	−	+
M. ovipneumoniae	+	−	−	−	−	−	−
M. arginini	+	−	−	+	−	−	−
M. putrefaciens	+	−	+	−	+	+	−
M. conjunctivae	+	−	+	−	−	+	−
Taxon 2D	+	−	−	−	+	+	−
Taxon G	+	−	−	+	−	−	−
Taxon U	+	−	+	+	+	−	−
Taxon V	+	−	+	−	−	−	[b]
Ureaplasmas	+	+	−	−	−[b]	−	−
A. oculi	+	−	+	−	−	−	−
A. laidlawii	−	−	+	−	−	−	−

Note: Definitive identification is done with fluorescent antibody tests or growth inhibition test using antisera raised against type strains.
[a] Some strains may be negative even after prolonged incubation.
[b] No available data.

taxon. Experimentally, the LC-type is very virulent, causing pleuropneumonia and septicemia in goats and sheep exposed to a respiratory challenge; but it is less contagious than CCPP.

The LC-type grows rapidly on Hayflick's medium. The inexperienced may mistake the unusual turbidity in broth and the large colonies for bacterial contamination. Identification is based on the criteria in Table 7.2 followed by FA or GI test with serum against strain Y–goat or any other recognized reference strain for this group.

It may be possible to recognize mycoplasmas in direct smears of joint exudate, mammary secretions, and pleural fluid by May-Grünwald-Giemsa staining or dark-field microscopy. It may also be worthwhile to use the acridine orange staining technique for this purpose.

Specific polysaccharide antigen produced by the mycoplasma may be detected in extracts of inflamed tissue by the gel precipitation test.[17]

The CF and indirect hemagglutination (IHA) tests have been used for serodiagnosis of infections with the LC-type and appear to be useful for herd diagnosis, but are not sufficiently reliable for individual diagnosis.[25]

Mycoplasma mycoides subspecies *capri* (*M. capri*)

M. capri has many features in common with the LC-type although significant surface antigens are different. This organism is also specific for goats and may cause septicemia and various local manifestations, such as polyarthritis. It may be isolated from the lungs of cases loosely diagnosed as CCPP but, although highly virulent under experimental conditions, it is not considered the primary cause of "classical" CCPP.[21] The approach to isolation and identification of *M. capri* is similar to the LC-type. Serological diagnosis of infection may be attempted with IHA or CF test, but more modern tests such as ELISA may be just as useful and less cumbersome.[13]

Mycoplasma capricolum

Infections with *M. capricolum* occur in both sheep and goats. The organism is highly invasive and may cause outbreaks similar to the contagious agalactia syndrome and the septicemic disease seen with the LC-type. Fatal septicemia-polyarthritis may occur in kids or lambs fed contaminated milk from dams with *M. capricolum* mastitis. Sporadic arthritis and abscesses may be less serious manifestations of *M. capricolum* infection.[24]

The organism grows readily on Hayflick's medium and is identified according to Table 7.2 and results of FA or GI. Reported serodiagnostic tests include CF and IHA.

Taxon F-38

The group of mycoplasmas identical with strain F-38 are now believed to be responsible for the "classical" CCPP. Some of the isolates in taxon F-38 are related to *M. capricolum,* which has caused some hesitation in designating the taxon as a new species.[4] Taxon F-38 appears to be more fastidious than strains of *M. capricolum, M. capri,* or the LC-type, and should be isolated on MacOwans VFG medium[17] or the medium formulated according to Jones and Wood[17] (see appendix at the end of this chapter). It is recommended to use the dilution technique and broth enrichment in order to increase the chance of successful isolation. Tissue samples should be minced, but not ground or homogenized, in broth and serially diluted to 10^{-4}. Aliquots from the suspension and the dilutions should be plated immediately and after 4 and 8 days, or if color changes or turbidity occur. Suspected F-38 isolates should be examined biochemically (Table 7.2) and serologically. Cross-reactivity should be expected in FA, GI, and growth precipitation tests with *M. capricolum* and the bovine taxon "Group 7." Until more specific reagents such as monoclonal antibodies are available, it may not be possible to arrive at a definitive diagnosis.

Goat sera have been examined for antibodies against F-38 with CF and IHA tests, but more information is needed on the diagnostic sensitivity and specificity of these tests.[14,22]

Mycoplasma ovipneumoniae

M. ovipneumoniae is a proven pathogen of sheep, which acts in concert with *Pasteurella haemolytica* to cause proliferative exudative pneumonia.[29,30] Whether viruses contribute to this form of pneumonia is uncertain. *M. ovipneumoniae* is recovered frequently from the respiratory tract of goats, but its contribution to lung pathology in this host species is not clear. Challenge experiments have shown that *M. ovipneumoniae* is capable of causing pneumonia and extensive fibrinous pleuritis in goats, but there seems to be considerable variation in susceptibility.[10] More strains of *M. ovipneumoniae* need to be examined. *M. ovipneumoniae* is present in the naso-pharyngeal cavity and must be recovered from lung tissue or bronchoalveolar lavage fluid of pneumonic animals for the diagnosis to be meaningful. *M. ovipneumoniae* is relatively fastidious and is best isolated using the dilution technique and the modified Friis' medium[8,17] (see appendix at the end of this chapter). Colonies appear after 4–8 days, but lack the typical "fried egg" morphology. The colony morphology and requirement for special media together with source of sample strongly indicate the identity, which may only need to be confirmed by GI. It is difficult to identify

M. ovipneumoniae by FA because the colonies tend to wash off the agar since they lack the ability to grow into the agar. The colony blotting technique described by Kotani and McGarrity may be well suited for serological identification of *M. ovipneumoniae*.[15] The IHA test is useful for serodiagnosis of *M. ovipneumoniae* infections.[10]

Mycoplasma arginini

This species is frequently recovered from the respiratory and genital tracts and eyes, but its pathogenicity is probably insignificant. *M. arginini* is not specific for sheep and goats. It is isolated and identified by standard procedures. Goats challenged experimentally respond with antibodies detectable by IHA.[10]

Mycoplasma putrefaciens

This mycoplasma has been associated with mastitis-agalactia in goats.[1,9] A dairy herd in California experienced a severe outbreak of *M. putrefaciens* infection affecting almost all the animals. The does developed mastitis and arthritis and the kids septicemia with arthritis. The infection apparently spread via contaminated milking equipment and contaminated colostrum and milk fed to the kids.[6] Under laboratory conditions 50 organisms cause clinical mastitis in some goats and subclinical infection in others. *M. putrefaciens* may be isolated from milk samples and joint taps using Hayflick's medium, and identified according to the characteristics in Table 7.2. Both agar and broth cultures of *M. putrefaciens* produce a putrid odor unusual for mycoplasmas. Tube agglutination (TA) and CF tests may be used for serodiagnosis.

Mycoplasma conjunctivae

Infectious keratoconjunctivitis ("pinkeye") is a disease of worldwide distribution of sheep and goats.[31] If *M. conjunctivae* is introduced by a carrier animal into a herd of immunologically naive animals, the infection spreads rapidly resulting in an outbreak of keratoconjunctivitis. The signs include conjunctivitis, keratitis, and increased lacrimation, but the disease tends to be self-limiting after a course of 2–3 weeks, and permanent corneal lesions are rare; the occurrence of corneal ulceration is thought to be due to secondary bacterial infection.

M. conjunctivae is most conveniently isolated on Hayflick's agar from eye or nasal swabs and identified by standard techniques. Antibodies in infected animals may be detected by metabolism inhibition test (MIT).

Taxon 2D

Mycoplasmas identical with strain 2D have been isolated from the genital tract of sheep with vulvovaginitis and reproductive problems.[20] Strains in this taxon are apparently related to *M. agalactiae* and *M. mycoides,* but the definitive taxonomical affiliation has not been established. Taxon 2D strains grow well on Hayflick's medium and should be identified according to the biochemical characteristics in Table 7.2 and positive FA or GI reactions with antiserum against strain 2D.

Taxons G,U,V

Mycoplasmas which appear to be antigenically different from established species have been isolated from the external ear canal of goats.[5] A few strains of these unclassified taxons have been isolated from other sites, but their role in disease conditions is not clear.

Acholeplasma oculi

This *Acholeplasma* species may be a contributing factor in keratoconjunctivitis.[2] It is often isolated together with *M. conjunctivae* and has been shown to cause keratoconjunctivitis by itself in experimentally inoculated goats.

Hayflick's medium is satisfactory for isolating *A. oculi* from nasal samples or eye swabs. Digitonin resistance identifies the isolate in the genus *Acholeplasma,* and should be followed by FA or GI tests with antiserum against the type strain of *A. oculi.*

Acholeplasma laidlawii

This organism is not host specific and may frequently be isolated from both sheep and goats, but should generally be ruled out as a pathogen.

Ureaplasmas

Ureaplasmas are readily isolated from the urogenital tract and occasionally from the respiratory tract of sheep and goats. Their role in disease is not clear, but the diagnostician may consider them significant in cases of infertility, abortion, and birth of weak lambs or kids in which ureaplasmas are cultured in abundance in the absence of other obvious pathogenic microorganisms.[19] There is some evidence to suggest that ureaplasmas may be responsible for certain cases of urinary calculi in goats on a low calcium diet, but the significance of this problem on a wider scale needs to be evaluated.[18] They may also cause a mild vulvovaginitis.[3]

Ureaplasmas require special media, such as the one formulated by Livingston or Jones[12] (See appendix), and are easily recognized on the basis of rapid growth, preferred anaerobic atmosphere, and urease activity. It is not necessary to go beyond biochemical identification because no widely accepted serotyping scheme is as yet established for ovine and caprine ureaplasmas. The immune response to ureaplasmas is relatively poor in field cases, making serodiagnosis very difficult. A recently developed ELISA technique using ureaplasma antigen immobilized on nitrocellulose paper may be useful.[16]

References

1. Adler HE, DaMassa AJ, Brooks DL: 1980, Caprine mycoplasmosis: *Mycoplasma putrefaciens,* a new cause of mastitis in goats. Am J Vet Res 41:1677–1679.

2. Arbuckle JBR, Bonson MD: 1980, The isolation of *Acholeplasma oculi* from an outbreak of ovine keratoconjunctivitis. Vet Rec 106:15.

3. Ball HJ, McCaughey WJ: 1982, Experimental production of vulvitis in ewes with a ureaplasma isolate. Vet Rec 110:581.

4. Christiansen C and Ernø H: 1982, Classification of the F-38 group of caprine mycoplasma strains by DNA hybridization. J Gen Microbiol 128:2523–2526.

5. Cottew GS, Yeats FR: 1982, Mycoplasmas and mites in the ears of clinically normal goats. Aust Vet J 59:77–81.

6. DaMassa AJ, Brooks DL, Holmberg CA, Moe AI: 1987, Caprine mycoplasmosis: An outbreak of mastitis and arthritis requiring the destruction of 700 goats. Vet Rec 120:409–413.

7. East NE, DaMassa AJ, Logan LL, Brooks DL, McGowan B: 1983, Milkborne outbreak of *Mycoplasma mycoides* subspecies *mycoides* infection in a commercial goat dairy. J Am Vet Med Assoc 182:1338–1341.

8. Friis NF: 1974, Mycoplasmas in pigs with special regard to the respiratory tract. Commissioned by: DSR Forlag Royal Veterinary and Agricultural University, Copenhagen.

9. Gaillard-Perrin G, Picavet DP, Perrin G: 1985, Isolement de *Mycoplasma putrefaciens* dans deux troupeaux de chèvres présentant des symptomes d'agalactie. Revue Med Vet 137:67–70.

10. Goltz JP, Rosendal S, McCraw BM, Ruhnke HL: 1986, Experimental studies on the

pathogenicity of *Mycoplasma ovipneumoniae* and *Mycoplasma arginini* for the respiratory tract of goats. Can J Vet Res 50:59–67.

11. Jasper DE, Rosendal S, Barnum DA: 1984, Acridine orange staining for diagnosis of *Mycoplasma bovis* infection in cow milk. J Clin Microb 20:624–625.

12. Jones GE: 1978, Studies on mycoplasmas of the respiratory tract of sheep. Ph.D. thesis, University of Edinburgh, 270 pp.

13. Jones GE ed: 1987, Contagious agalactia and other mycoplasmal diseases of small ruminants. Agricultural Commission of the European Communities. Sept. 19–20, 1985, Nice, France.

14. Jones GE, Wood AR: 1988, Microbiological and serological studies on caprine pneumonias in Oman. Res Vet Sci 44:125–131.

15. Kotani H, McGarrity GJ: 1985, Rapid and simple identification of mycoplasmas by immunobinding. J Immun Methods 85:257–267.

16. Kreplin CMA: 1988, A study of infertility and the immune response associated with *Ureaplasma diversum* infection in cattle. Ph.D. thesis, University of Guelph, 298 pp.

17. Lefevre PC, Jones GE, Ojo MO: 1987, Pulmonary mycoplasmosis of small ruminants. Rev Sci Tech Off Int Epiz 6:759–799.

18. Livingston CW Jr, Calhoun MC, Gauer BB, Baldwin BC Jr: 1984, Effect of experimental infection with ovine ureaplasma upon the development of uroliths in feedlot lambs. Israel J Med Sci 20:958–961.

19. Livingston CW Jr, Gauer BB: 1982, Effect of venereal transmission of ovine ureaplasma on reproductive efficiency of ewes. Am J Vet Res 43:1190–1193.

20. Livingston CW Jr, Gauer BB: 1983, Occurrence of *Mycoplasma* sp. (2D) in Texas sheep flocks. Am J Vet Res 44:868–869.

21. McMartin DA, MacOwan KJ, Swift LL: 1980, A century of classical contagious caprine pleuropneumonia: from original description to aetiology. Br Vet J 136:507–515.

22. Muthomi EK, Rurangirwa FR: 1983, Passive haemagglutination and complement fixation as diagnostic tests for contagious caprine pleuropneumonia caused by the F-38 strain of mycoplasma. Res Vet Sci 35:1–4.

23. Perreau P: 1979, Les mycoplasmoses de la chèvre. Cah Med Vet 48:71–85.

24. Perreau P, Breard A: 1979, La mycoplasmose caprine à *M. capricolum*. Comp Immun Microbiol Infect Dis 2:87–97.

25. Rosendal S: 1983, Susceptibility of goats and calves after experimental inoculation or contact exposure to a Canadian strain of *Mycoplasma mycoides* subsp. *mycoides* isolated from a goat. Can J Comp Med 47:484–490.

26. Ruhnke HL, Rosendal S, Goltz J, Blackwell TE: 1983, Isolation of *Mycoplasma mycoides* subspecies *mycoides* from polyarthritis and mastitis of goats in Canada. Can Vet J 24:54–56.

27. Schaeren von W, Nicolet J: 1982, Anwendung eines Micro-ELISA für die Serologie der infektiosen Agalaktie der Ziegen. Schweiz Arch Tierheilk 124:163–177.

28. Singh N, Rajya BS, Mohanty GC: 1975, Pathology of *Mycoplasma agalactiae* induced granular vulvovaginitis (GVV) in goats. Cornell Vet 65:363–373.

29. Sullivan ND, St. George TD, Horsfall N: 1973, A proliferative interstitial pneumonia of sheep associated with mycoplasma infection: 1. Natural history of the disease in a flock. Aust Vet J 49:57–62.

30. Sullivan ND, St. George TD, Horsfall N: 1973, A proliferative interstitial pneumonia of sheep associated with mycoplasma infection: 2. The experimental exposure of young lambs to infection. Aust Vet J 49:63–68.

31. Trotter SL, Franklin RM, Baas EJ, Barile MF: 1977, Epidemic caprine keratoconjunctivitis: Experimentally induced disease with a pure culture of *Mycoplasma conjunctivae*. Infect and Immun 18:816–822.

Appendix A7.1

WJB Medium[17]
Autoclaved portion
  Bacto PPLO broth base w/o crystal violet
    (Difco Laboratories, Detroit, MI)   1.5 g
  Bacto-tryptone (Difco)   1.5 g
  Bacto-peptone (Difco)   0.3 g
  Bacto-yeast-extract (Difco)   0.1 g
  Deionized water   50.0 ml

Membrane filtered components		
Newborn calf serum (inactivated)	45.0	ml
10 × Medium 199 without NaHCO$_3$, with		
glutamine (Gibco)	5.0	ml
Fresh yeast extract	5.0	ml
Calf thymus DNA (highly polymerized; 0.2% w/v)	1.0	ml
Glucose (50% w/v)	0.5	ml
NADH (10% w/v)	0.1	ml
Ampicillin (100 mg/ml)	0.25	ml
Thallous acetate (10% w/v)	0.25	ml
Phenol red (0.4% w/v)	1.5	ml

Adjusted to pH 7.6–7.8 with 1 M NaOH.
Solid medium: Add 0.9% agarose.

Modified Friis' Medium[8]
Autoclaved portion

10 × Hanks' balanced salt solution	3.0	ml
Deionized water	72.0	ml
Bacto-brain-heart infusion (Difco)	0.5	g
Mycoplasma broth base (BBL Microbiology Systems)	0.75	g
Lactalbumin hydrolysate	0.125	g
Yeast-extract (Difco)	0.05	g
Phenol red (0.1% w/v) solution	1.37	ml

Membrane filtered components		
Fresh yeast extract (25% w/v)	3.65	ml
Glucose (50% w/v)	0.25	ml
Thallous acetate (2% w/v)	0.55	ml
Horse serum	10.0	ml
Swine serum (inactivated)	10.0	ml

Solid medium: Add 0.9% agarose.

Modified Hayflick's Medium[12]
Autoclaved portion

Bacto PPLO broth w/o crystal violet (Difco)	2.1	g
Deionized water	70.0	ml

Membrane filtered components

Newborn calf serum (inactivated)	20.0	ml
Fresh yeast extract	10.0	ml
Calf thymus DNA (highly polymerized; 0.2% w/v)	1.0	ml
Ampicillin (100 mg/ml)	0.25	ml
Thallous acetate (10% w/v)	0.25	ml
Triphenyl tetrazolium chloride (2% w/v)	1.0	ml

Adjusted to pH 7.6–7.8 with 1 M NaOH.

Solid medium: Use Bacto PPLO agar w/o crystal violet instead of Bacto PPLO broth in the amount recommended by the manufacturer.

TB Medium (Ureaplasmas)[18]

10 × Medium 199	4.8	ml
Hartley's digest broth	20.0	ml
Fresh yeast extract	10.0	ml
Inactivated pig serum	20.0	ml
Urea (20% w/v)	0.5	ml
Calf thymus DNA (0.2% w/v)	1.0	ml
Dithiothreitol (10% w/v)	1.0	ml
Ampicillin (100 mg/ml)	0.25	ml
Thallium acetate (10% w/v)	0.25	ml
Phenol red (0.4% w/v)	1.5	ml
Deionized water	40.0	ml
Adjust pH to 6.0.		

Solid medium: Add 0.9% agarose.

Livingston's Medium (Ureaplasmas)

Trypsin digested beef heart infusion (20%)	100.0	ml
NaCl solution (1% w/v)	100.0	ml
Glucose	0.2	g
Autoclave and adjust pH to 6.0.		

Add:

Horse serum	58.0	ml
Fresh yeast extract	29.0	ml
Urea solution (10% w/v)	0.7	ml

Phenol red solution	0.3 ml
CVA enrichment	1.0 ml
L-cysteine hydrochloride solution (4% w/v)	0.5 ml
MnSO$_4$ solution (0.1% w/v)	3.0 ml

Solid medium: Add 1.0% Ionagar.

Direct Demonstration of Mycoplasmas in Mastitis

Acridine orange is dissolved in phosphate-citrate buffer (pH 3.0) to make a 0.01% solution, which can be stored, protected from light, at 4°C for 6 months.

Milk secretions, perhaps clarified by brief centrifugation at 1000 × G for 5 minutes, are mixed in equal volumes with acridine orange solution and allowed to stand for a few minutes. Ten microliters of the mixture are placed on an agar plate and covered with a coverslip. The preparation is examined with a microscope with epifluorescence equipment. Mycoplasmas fluoresce bright green and are usually round or slightly elongated. Bacteria also fluoresce, but are larger and have a distinctive morphology and arrangement according to group. If the milk sample appears normal it may be difficult to recognize mycoplasmas because of the many fat globules, but in the more or less clear whey formed on top of a mastitis sample this is not a problem.

Mycoplasmas of Laboratory Rodents

M. K. DAVIDSON
J. K. DAVIS
G. P. GAMBILL
G. H. CASSELL
J. R. LINDSEY

Numerous species of mycoplasmas have been isolated from rodents;[9,39] most are considered commensals, although this judgment is often based solely on failure to produce grossly evident disease. Both the pathogenic and nonpathogenic species of mycoplasmas of rats and mice are listed in Table 8.1. Other laboratory rodents also have mycoplasmas, but we will address only the diagnosis of mycoplasmal infections in rats and mice. Currently, rats and mice are the only species in which mycoplasmal disease is a well-recognized problem,[4,9,39,41] and the techniques and media that are used for rats and mice can be used for the recovery of mycoplasmas from other rodent species.

Experimental animals free of indigenous pathogens are essential to the production of accurate, reproducible research data. Obviously, morbidity and mortality resulting from infectious agents can drastically affect research. Not as obvious, but of equal concern, are the consequences of subclinical infections that can affect the validity of data without the investi-

This work was supported by Public Health Service grants RR00959 and RR00463 from the Division of Research Resources, National Institutes of Health, and funds from the Veterans Administration Research Service.

Table 8.1.   Mycoplasmas isolated from rats and mice

Mycoplasma Species	Natural Host(s)	Metabolism	Frequency of Infection	Natural Disease
M. pulmonis	Rats, Mice	Glucose	Common	Yes
M. arthritidis	Rats, Mice	Arginine	Common	Yes[a]
M. neurolyticum	Mice	Glucose	Rare	No
M. collis	Rats, Mice	Glucose	Unknown	Unknown
M. muris	Mice	Arginine	Unknown	Unknown
KE2	Rats	Glucose, arginine	Unknown	Unknown

[a]Natural disease has been reported, but it is extremely rare.

gator even being aware that an infectious agent is present.[8,37,39,41] There is substantial evidence that subclinical infections with *Mycoplasma pulmonis* or *Mycoplasma arthritidis* have interfered with a wide variety of studies.[10,40,41] A classical example is the production of lung cancer by N-nitroso-heptamethylenimine. Tumor incidence increased from less than 20% in male rats free of *M. pulmonis* to more than 80% in infected males.[57]

Undoubtedly, the rodent mycoplasmas continue to affect the validity of research data. Rats and mice are the most common animals used for research in the United States, with approximately 18 million used annually.[35] Of these, approximately 65% of the mice and 81% of the rats are produced in commercial breeding facilities.[36,38] Even in these so-called "barrier" breeding facilities, a wide range of pathogens, including mycoplasmas, have been found in high prevalence.[4,8,36,38,41] In the early 1980's, serologic methods indicated that 91% of barrier-maintained mouse colonies and 78% of barrier-maintained rat colonies contained animals that were infected by one or more species of mycoplasmas.[11,36] There is little reason to believe that the situation is dramatically improved today.

Prevalence and Disease

Mycoplasma pulmonis

By far, the most important mycoplasma found in rats and mice is *M. pulmonis,* the etiologic agent of murine respiratory mycoplasmosis (MRM).[9,10,39–41] Virtually all conventional rat and mouse colonies in the United States are infected with this organism,[4,8,36,38,41] and the prevalence of *M. pulmonis* in animals within commercial barrier colonies is estimated to be 19% for mice and 17% for rats.[38] These estimates are based on cultural isolation from a single site, a notoriously insensitive method.[7,11,18] Therefore, the true prevalence is probably at least 5–10% higher.

MRM varies greatly in expression because of environmental, host, and mycoplasmal factors that influence the host-parasite relationship.[9,10,39–41]

Factors that are known to influence disease expression include environmental NH_3[1,53,54] or NO_2;[47] concurrent infections with either cilia-associated respiratory (CAR) bacillus,[25,41] Sendai virus,[52,55] or sialodacryoadenitis virus;[56] genetic susceptibility of the host;[20,22] and virulence of the organism.[19] However, *M. pulmonis* infection occurs most commonly without clinical signs, and under ideal conditions for the host, the organism causes minimal lesions.[4,7,8,11,18,41] Clinical signs, when present, are nonspecific, but may include "snuffling" (in rats), "chattering" (in mice), rales, polypnea, weight loss, hunched posture, ruffled coat, inactivity, "head tilt," and, in rats, accumulation of porphyrin pigment around the eyes and external nares.[10,39,40]

M. pulmonis preferentially colonizes the luminal surface of respiratory epithelium. Organisms (and lesions, if present) tend to decrease from proximal to distal airways. Characteristic lesions of MRM at any level of the respiratory tract include: neutrophils in the airways, hyperplasia of mucosal epithelium, and a lymphoid response in the submucosa. Lesions may be acute or chronic and include: rhinitis, otitis media, laryngitis, tracheitis, bronchitis, bronchiectasis, pulmonary abscesses, and alveolitis.[39] Pleuritis and emphysema are rare. There is dramatic hyperplasia of bronchus-associated lymphoid tissue in rats.[10,39] Syncytial giant cells may occur in the epithelium of the nasal and bronchial mucosa in mice.[39,40]

Natural infections of *M. pulmonis* also occur in the genital tract of rats.[39,41] In addition to increased severity of MRM,[20] rats of the LEW strain, at least, are highly susceptible to severe genital disease characterized by purulent endometritis or pyometra, salpingitis and perioophoritis.[41]

Mycoplasma arthritidis

Based on cultural isolation, 3% of the barrier-maintained mouse colonies and 6% of the barrier-maintained rat colonies have been found to be infected with *M. arthritidis*.[38] However, these data are deceiving. Subclinical infections with *M. arthritidis* are very difficult to demonstrate culturally. Immunologic methods of diagnosis suggest that *M. arthritidis* is common in contemporary rat and mouse populations, and may actually be the most common of the murine mycoplasmas.[4,36,38]

The literature contains less than a dozen reports of natural arthritis due to *M. arthritidis* in rats, the most recent dated 1969.[14] Other reports of natural infections in rats have appeared infrequently since 1938.[41] Most of the recent literature concerns laboratory models of arthritis produced by inoculating large doses of *M. arthritidis* intravenously or into the footpads of mice.[41] Natural infections in mice were first reported in 1983.[17] In that study, organisms were isolated from the nasal passages, conjunctiva, laryngo-tracheo-bronchial system (by lavage), and the uterus. However, no

gross or microscopic lesions attributable to the mycoplasma were found.[17]
Current evidence suggests that subclinical *M. arthritidis* infection occurs in many colonies of rats and mice.[4,36,38] The preferred host sites and natural history of these infections are unknown. Lesions are not present in subclinical infections. The pathology of the experimental arthritis in rats and mice due to *M. arthritidis* has been reviewed by Lindsey et al.[38]

Mycoplasma neurolyticum

M. neurolyticum has been isolated occasionally from mice and rats since 1938,[41] but there has been only one instance in which it was thought to be a natural pathogen. Nelson[9,44] described a colony of mice in which he associated the occurrence of conjunctivitis with the presence of this organism. This has not been confirmed, and experimental inoculations into mice have failed to cause disease.[9] Thus, this organism is considered a commensal. It has been isolated from the conjunctiva, nasal passages, Harderian glands, and brain of laboratory mice, and from the conjunctiva of laboratory rats.[9] *M. neurolyticum* may be common in conventional rat and mouse colonies, but the prevalence in barrier-maintained stocks appears to be very low since it is rarely isolated, even by laboratories that routinely culture for the organism using suitable media.

No gross or microscopic lesions are associated with natural infections or experimental inoculations into the conjunctiva or nasal passages.[9,39] The organism produces a thermolabile, neurotoxic endotoxin which causes "rolling disease" in mice or young rats.[9,39,40] This experimentally-induced disease causes severe cerebral edema manifested clinically by rolling from side to side.[39,40] There is extreme distension of astrocytes by fluid; mechanical displacement, compression, and degeneration of myelinated axons; and accumulation of extracellular fluid in the white matter.[9,39,40]

Mycoplasma collis

This organism has been isolated from one mouse colony and four rat colonies in the United Kingdom. The organism was recovered from the conjunctiva of mice,[9,29] and the conjunctiva, Harderian gland, and nasopharynx in rats.[9,29] Infected rats had conjunctivitis, but attempts to reproduce the disease in pathogen-free rats failed.[9,29] Clinical signs have not been observed in infected mice.[9,29] The organism is considered a commensal, and the prevalence is unknown.

Mycoplasma muris **and KE2**

M. muris, an anaerobic mycoplasma, has been isolated from the vagina of pregnant RIII mice,[43] and KE2 has been isolated from the colon and cecum of wild rats in Germany.[27] Attempts to isolate the latter from laboratory rats have failed[33] (H. Kirchhoff, personal communication), and neither organism has been associated with disease. The prevalence of both is unknown.

Diagnosis of Mycoplasmal Infections

Diagnosis of murine mycoplasmas in clinically ill animals is not difficult, and any of the procedures listed below will suffice. However, in well-managed animal facilities, clinically ill animals are rare. The diagnostic challenges are: (a) the detection of subclinical infections which often have very small numbers of organisms present and (b) differentiation of the pathogenic mycoplasmal species from those that are currently considered commensals.

Health surveillance programs should be designed to give at least a 95% chance of detecting at least one infected animal at a given prevalence of infection. The sample size (number of animals) to be tested is of critical importance and can be determined mathematically if a truly random sample can be obtained, the prevalence of the infection is known or can be estimated, and **the detection method approximates 100% accuracy.**[5,15] As shown in Table 8.2, if one assumes that 40% of the animals in a population are infected with an agent, there is a 99% probability that one infected animal will be detected in a random sample of ten animals. This approximates detection of *M. pulmonis* in many well-managed conventional rodent colonies. However, to detect one infected animal in a population with a 1% prevalence rate would require testing a random sample of over 200 animals.[15] Unfortunately, the latter situation more accurately describes the chance of detecting infection without specialized cultural or ancillary techniques in colonies of "cesarian-derived, barrier-maintained" rodents. Since

Table 8.2. Minimal number of samples needed to detect infections

Incidence of Infection (%)	Sample Size Necessary for Confidence Limit	
	95%	99%
5	60	90
10	29	44
15	19	24
20	14	21
25	11	16
30	9	13
40	6	9
50	5	7

Note: Table shows the minimum number of animals that must be sampled to detect infectious agents at the indicated prevalence rates within the population. Samples must be taken with complete randomization from a population of 100 or more animals. The disease must show no age or sex predilection.

diagnosis of infection in these colonies is much more difficult than in heavily infected populations, we will direct our discussion to the former on the premise that techniques that work for these colonies also will work in the more heavily infected populations.

Histopathology

Gross lung lesions are inconsistent in MRM, even in infected conventional animals. Only in old animals, animals of highly susceptible strains (LEW rats or C3H/HeN mice), or in animals experimentally inoculated with large doses of *M. pulmonis,* are characteristic gross lesions common. Examination of lungs and nasal passages for microscopic lesions is much more useful. However, even microscopic lesions are rare or minimal in animals infected with low numbers of organisms. Thus, histopathology is insensitive and requires special training to interpret the results. Mild infections are easily overlooked unless one studies multiple tissues and is very familiar with minor changes in rat or mouse tissues. In addition, lesions are usually not diagnostic, just suggestive of possible diagnoses. Reviews of the disease and lesions of MRM have been published previously.[10,39,40] Natural infections with *M. arthritidis* or *M. neurolyticum* usually do not produce lesions, and the recently isolated species appear to be commensals. Lesions have not been recognized for infections with *M. collis, M. muris,* or KE2.

Detection of Mycoplasmal Antigen in Tissues

Immunofluorescence and immunoperoxidase methods for detection of mycoplasmal antigen in tissues have been described,[10,18,28,37,40,42] and both work well in animals that are heavily infected. However, they usually require special processing of the tissues[28,40,51] and experienced personnel to interpret the results. As we have demonstrated with experimentally infected animals, the ability to detect *M. pulmonis* in tissues is directly related to the number of organisms present.[18] In animals infected with 10^3 CFU or less, immunofluorescence detected less than 50% of infected animals, and even this degree of success required examination of the trachea, larynx, and lungs. Examination of a single site gave a much lower success rate. In addition, following low-dose experimental inoculation, the majority of *M. pulmonis* organisms localized in the nasal passages,[18] a site notoriously difficult to examine by immunofluorescence. Decalcification is required before sectioning of the nasal passages, and *M. pulmonis* antigen often is not detectable following this procedure. In addition, the organism usually can be cultivated readily from animals that are positive by immunofluorescence.[40]

Culture

GENERAL RECOMMENDATIONS

Murine mycoplasmas have been isolated from a wide variety of anatomical sites. There is general agreement that *M. pulmonis* most frequently inhabits the upper respiratory tract and the middle ear. However, since mycoplasmas have been isolated from so many different sites, there is controversy concerning the best *single* site for optimal recovery.[5,18] In general, it is recommended that multiple sites be sampled for cultural isolation of all murine mycoplasmas.[4-6,18] Any sampling strategy should include at least one site in the respiratory tract. Identification of isolates must conform to the standards adopted by the Subcommittee on the Taxonomy of the Mollicutes.[23,31] The characteristics listed in Table 8.3 are helpful, but final identification should be based upon growth inhibition,[13] immunofluorescence,[26] or immunoperoxidase[48] staining with specific antisera.

Table 8.3.   Differential features of known murine mycoplasmas

Species	Glucose Catabolism	Arginine Hydrolysis	Hemad-sorption[a]	Tetrazolium Reduction	Resazurin Reduction
M. pulmonis	+	−	+	variable	+
M. arthritidis	−	+	−	−	−
M. neurolyticum	+	−	−	−	−
M. collis[b]	+	−	+	+	+
M. muris[c]	−	+	+	+	ND[d]
KE2[e]	+	+	ND	−	ND

[a] Guinea pig red blood cells.
[b] Additional biochemical tests are needed to distinguish between *M. pulmonis* and *M. collis*.[29]
[c] This organism is a strict anaerobe. All tests were done under anaerobic conditions.[42]
[d] Not done.
[e] This organism recently has been isolated from wild rats by Giebel et al.,[27] and has not yet been completely characterized.

Proper specimen collection is as important as preparation and quality control of the medium (see Appendix A8.2 at the end of this chapter for a discussion of quality control of media). Mycoplasmas usually inhabit mucosal surfaces and are often unevenly dispersed within organ systems. Therefore, lavage is one of the better sampling techniques. Swabbing also works well, but is better suited for organs, such as the larynx. One should concentrate on sites with active disease, exudates, or increased mucus. Tissue homogenates may be used for special procedures, such as quantitative cultures,[54] if measures are taken to avoid the effects of tissue inhibitors.[5,58]

Cultivation of mycoplasmas from clinically ill animals is generally not difficult assuming the proper selection of sites to be cultured, collection of an adequate sample, and pretesting of the medium to assure its ability to support growth. Most murine mycoplasmas will grow in standard Hay-flick's medium[24] or in SP4 medium,[61] but we have found the formulation of Medium A (see Appendix A8.1 at the end of this chapter) to be superior to other media for *M. pulmonis, M. arthritidis, M. neurolyticum,* and *M. collis. M. muris* grows best in SP4 medium.[43] Because this organism is a strict anaerobe, the medium must be prereduced. Placing the medium in an anaerobe jar (GasPak anaerobe system, BBL Microbiology Systems, Cock-eysville, MD) overnight is usually sufficient.

We prefer cefoperazone to other antimicrobial agents because this drug is bacteriocidal to most walled bacteria, including highly resistant *Pseudomonas* sp. and enterococci, which are common inhabitants of the intestinal tract of rats and mice. Since rats and mice are coprophagic, these organisms frequently contaminate the upper respiratory tract and oral cavity. Cefoperazone does not harm or inhibit the growth of any of the murine mycoplasmal strains we have tested. If other antimicrobial agents are used in lieu of cefoperazone, pretesting of the medium with all of the mycoplasmas of interest is mandatory because some antimicrobial agents are inhibitory for some species but not for others. For example, some strains of *M. neurolyticum* are inhibited by penicillin.[24]

All of the murine mycoplasmas require a humid environment (90–95% relative humidity). Although some investigators strongly recommend an atmosphere with an elevated CO_2 content for mycoplasma isolation, all of the murine species except *M. muris* seem to grow better in room air than in 5–15% CO_2. However, mycoplasmas have been isolated from a wide variety of body sites, and different strains may be adapted to sites with an elevated CO_2 concentration. Therefore, if isolation of mycoplasmas from unusual anatomical sites is desired, inclusion of a 5–15% CO_2 atmosphere in the cultural protocol may be useful.

Mycoplasmas are very sensitive to drying so all swabs must be placed immediately into mycoplasmal broth. Lavage samples also should be placed as soon as possible into broth. Tissue samples contain mycoplasma-cidal substances, which may be inhibited by inclusion of ammonium reine-chate or lysophospholipase in the medium.[58] Alternatively, samples containing blood, purulent exudate, or tissue may be serially diluted by tenfold dilutions (10^{-1}–10^{-6}). All dilutions should be incubated; frequently only one tube will have obvious growth. In addition, each dilution should be plated on agar because some isolates prefer solid medium to broth. Some agars are inhibitory to mycoplasmas, so SeaPlaque agarose (FMC Biopro-ducts, Rockland, ME) is recommended for primary isolation of mycoplas-mas from animals. Although the common murine mycoplasmas usually grow within 1 week, all cultures should be incubated for at least 21 days before discarding as negative. Blind passages of cultures to broth and agar every 2 days will occasionally increase isolation rates.

MATERIALS

The following items are recommended for aseptic collection of samples from various body sites during health surveillance testing:

1. Sterile surgical instrument pack: 2″ × 2″ gauze sponges; 4″ × 4″ gauze sponges; "mosquito" hemostats; straight Mayo scissors; suture wire scissors; iris scissors; Adson forceps; and dissecting pins.
2. Dissecting board, covered with an absorbent pad.
3. Glass beakers for absolute alcohol and water. The alcohol is for sterilization of instruments. The water is for washing instruments between samples.
4. Alcohol burner or Bunsen burner.
5. Wash bottle filled with absolute alcohol.
6. Tissue grinders, i.e., mortar and pestle or tissue homogenizers.
7. Nasopharyngeal/urethral swabs, calcium alginate, sterile, type 1 (Inolex Corporation, Glenwood, IL).
8. Syringes, 1 cc, sterile, fitted with 18–25-gauge needles. Needle size varies with animal size and sample.
9. Sample collection fluid. Either sterile 0.85% NaCl (pyrogen-free, as for injection or IV fluid) or mycoplasma broth. Mycoplasmas will tolerate a short time in saline, if necessary. Specimens should be processed for culture within 30 minutes.
10. Tubes for blood collection.
11. Anesthetic. Some procedures can be done without anesthesia, but most sample collections in rodents require either euthanasia of the animal or surgical anesthesia. Sodium pentobarbital overdose may be used for euthanasia. A ketamine/xylazine combination provides good surgical anesthesia for rats and mice. Combine 150 mg of xylazine and 1000 mg ketamine. The dose for rats is 0.1 ml/100 g body weight, given intramuscularly (IM). For mice, dilute this preparation 1:10 in sterile water or 0.85% saline, then give 0.1 ml/ 20 g of body weight, IM.
12. Animal clippers (or razor blades for shaving fur) for hair removal. These are needed for collecting some specimens.

COLLECTION OF SPECIMENS FROM ANESTHETIZED ANIMALS

1. Nasal passage lavage. Use a tuberculin syringe and, depending on the size of the animal, an 18–22-gauge needle and 0.2–0.6 ml collection fluid. Insert the tip of the needle through the external nares and flush the fluid back and forth within the nasal passages, being careful not to damage the mucosa. Also, be careful not to flush too vigorously and lose fluid down the trachea or through the mouth.

2. Swabs. Cultures of the conjunctiva, oropharynx, vagina, or easily accessible sites may be taken with a nasopharyngeal/urethral swab.

COLLECTIONS OF SPECIMENS FROM ANIMALS AFTER EUTHANASIA

These procedures are designed for aseptic collection of comprehensive samples for culture with preservation of the tissues for other procedures, such as histology. Less complete protocols may be developed from these procedures. Animals should be humanely killed, preferably with an overdose of sodium pentobarbital. The animals should be exsanguinated when deep anesthesia is obtained. This decreases the chances of contaminating specimens with blood, which contains inhibitory substances. Place the animal on its back. The axillary or inguinal vessels may then be severed. The blood accumulates in the pocket formed between the leg and the body and can be collected or discarded, as desired. This blood collection method allows one to aseptically sample all body sites without contaminating the sites with invasive procedures (such as cardiac puncture). **Instruments must be sterilized between each step listed below by washing them with gauze and water, then dipping them in alcohol, and flaming.**

Respiratory tract

1. Clip the hair on the ventral surface from the chin to the pubis. This is not necessary if either a localized procedure is required, or the animal is thoroughly wet with absolute alcohol. (See 3, below.)
2. Place the animal on its back on a dissection board. Secure the feet. Dissection pins or rubber bands may be used to retract the feet and stretch the body.
3. Wet the entire ventral surface with absolute alcohol. A wash bottle works quite well for this. The alcohol prevents fur from contaminating the tissues and also disinfects the skin and fur.
4. Grasp the skin over the larynx with forceps and excise with scissors. Depending on the extent of the desired procedures, the skin may be removed from the entire ventral surface of the body. Do not penetrate the fascia. Wet the exposed area with alcohol.
5. Remove the submaxillary salivary glands, lymph nodes, and fat.
6. The thin omohyoid muscle can now be seen extending from the base of the tongue to the sternum. Remove the omohyoid muscle, thereby exposing the larynx and trachea.
7. Grasp the larynx and insert a needle through the tracheal wall, toward the lungs, to obtain a tracheobronchial lavage specimen. For an adult rat, use a 20-gauge needle on a tuberculin syringe containing 0.6 ml of collection fluid. For an adult mouse, use a 22-gauge needle and 0.4 ml collection fluid. Express and aspirate the fluid rather quickly while moving the bevel of the needle along the

interior tracheal wall. Repeat this 2–5 times. The volume of fluid recovered will vary considerably from animal to animal and with the experience of the collector. Greater volumes of fluid can be recovered by elevating the posterior part of the animal.

8. Remove the lower jaws. Carefully remove all soft tissues from the ventral portion of the larynx. Note the location of the soft palate.

9. Gently grasp the larynx with forceps and cut it free from the nasopharynx.

10. Swab the interior of the larynx with a nasopharyngeal/urethral swab.

11. Swab the interior of the nasopharynx with a nasopharyngeal/urethral swab. In rats, the swab can easily be inserted into the nasopharynx via the hole left when the larynx was cut from the soft palate. In mice, the soft palate will have to be cut longitudinally with iris scissors to allow entry of the swab. Alternatively, a lavage may be performed.

12. The tympanic bullae are exposed by removing the covering soft tissues. The bullae should be swabbed with alcohol and allowed to dry. Use a 22-gauge needle mounted on a tuberculin syringe to drill through the bullae into the middle ears. Lavage the middle ears with collection fluid.

13. An alternative culture sample that is satisfactory for most purposes is a lavage of the nasopharynx and the nasal passages. Remove the lower jaws as in step 8, then separate the head from the body by cutting through the spine at the cervical vertebrae. Clip off the soft tissues at the end of the nose to expose the bones slightly and eliminate contamination from the fur. Use a 22-gauge needle attached to a tuberculin syringe containing 1 ml of collection fluid. Place the end of the needle in the nasopharynx. Use forceps to place the head, nose down, over a sterile 12 × 75 mm test tube or other suitable collection vessel. Flush the collection fluid through the nasopharynx and nasal passages and collect the fluid in the test tube.

Genital tract

1. After removing the skin, wet the ventral abdominal wall with alcohol. Use forceps to lift the abdominal wall just anterior to the pubis, and cut with sterile scissors. Carefully transect the abdominal wall laterally and forward to the ribs. Reflect the abdominal wall, or remove it entirely.

2. Locate the genital tract by carefully retracting the intestines outside the abdominal cavity.

3. In females, a lavagate of the uterus and oviducts may be collected

in a tuberculin syringe with a 22–25-gauge needle and 0.3–0.5 ml collection fluid. Use mosquito hemostats to clamp the uterine horns at the cervix and the anterior end of each horn. Insert the needle between the clamps on each horn and gently lavage. A similar procedure may be used to collect amniotic fluid from pregnant females.

4. In males, swab the external urethral orifice with a nasopharyngeal/urethral swab and lavage the vas deferens with a tuberculin syringe with a 22–25-gauge needle and 0.3–0.5 ml collection fluid. If intact tissues are not needed for histology or other procedures, more accurate sampling is obtained by homogenizing each of the following tissues, either singly or in combination: preputial glands, testis, epididymis, prostate, vas deferens, coagulating gland, bladder, and urethra.

Other sites

1. *Joints.* Remove the skin and open the joint. Aseptically remove the synovium and cartilage. Alternatively, the joint may be swabbed or lavaged.

2. *Blood cultures.* It is virtually impossible to aseptically collect enough blood from an anesthetized animal for a blood culture. Blood obtained via orbital or tail bleeding is insufficient in volume and usually is contaminated. Therefore, give the animal enough ketamine/xylazine for euthanasia and, when the animal has reached the surgical plane of anesthesia, aseptically collect heart blood via cardiac puncture after the thoracic cavity is opened.

3. In addition to all of the previously mentioned sites, mycoplasmas can be recovered from the spleen, liver, brain, kidney, Harderian glands, and intestines of rats and mice. Any soft tissue may be aseptically collected and minced or homogenized.

LIMITATIONS

Isolation, cultivation, and positive identification of mycoplasmas by the above methods is difficult and may take 4 weeks or more. The media are expensive, and for animals from barrier-maintained colonies, multi-site samples are required. Even then, culture is relatively insensitive; up to 30% of pathogen-free rats experimentally infected with doses of 10^6 CFU of *M. pulmonis* were negative by culture at 28 days postinfection.[18] Since we do not know the natural sites of predilection for any of the murine mycoplasmas except *M. pulmonis,* it is impossible to know whether or not one has sampled a site that is likely to harbor organisms. In summary, culture is mandatory for verification of other methods, but is a poor screening technique because false negatives are common.

Enzyme-linked Immunosorbent Assay

BACKGROUND

Traditional methods of serologic diagnosis of mycoplasmal infections, such as complement fixation, hemagglutination, hemagglutination inhibition, and metabolic inhibition tests have been of little use in laboratory rodents because they are relatively insensitive and depend on antibody function. In well managed barrier-maintained rodent colonies, both the prevalence of infected animals and the numbers of organisms per animal are usually low. This situation makes detection by serologic methods very difficult. The enzyme-linked immunosorbent assay (ELISA) for mycoplasmal infections in rodents[3,30] has proven to be the best serologic test for screening large numbers of rodents. The test is relatively inexpensive to run, sensitive, rapid, and mycoplasmal genus-specific. In addition, animals do not have to be killed to obtain enough blood for the test. Blood may be collected from anesthetized animals by tail or orbital bleeding. However, the assay currently available cannot distinguish among mycoplasma species, and quality control of the assay, as with all serological assays, is critical for reliable results.

The techniques involved for the ELISA have been well described.[3,30] In its simplest form, the ELISA is performed by allowing mycoplasma antigen to adsorb nonspecifically to a solid phase (usually a 96-well microtiter plate), followed by sequential addition of the serum sample, the secondary conjugated antibody, and the enzyme substrate with adequate washing between reagent additions. The assay is completed by developing the colored product of the enzyme reaction, and reactions are read either on a spectrophotometer or by visual inspection. Although the "kit" form of the mycoplasmal ELISA is usually interpreted subjectively, the use of semi-quantitative data obtained by determining the intensity of the color change spectrophotometrically provides better discrimination of positive and negative results, which is especially important in monitoring barrier-maintained colonies. A semi-quantitative assay is relatively inexpensive and can easily be established in any laboratory with a spectrophotometer. However, different laboratories using this assay use different antigen preparations, different solid phase supports, different reagents, and variations in incubation times. All of these factors affect the test and have led to a lack of agreement in test results between different laboratories. Therefore, we will present the methods we have used to establish the particular set of conditions used in our assay. Since the ELISA for detection of *M. pulmonis* and the ELISAs for other murine mycoplasmas follow the original methods described by Horowitz and Cassell[30] and details of the methods are given elsewhere,[3,30] we will not discuss every detail of the entire test. It should be noted that high quality, commercially available, conjugated secondary antibodies, substrates, and developing reagents have eliminated the need for preparation of these reagents.

ANTIGEN PREPARATION

We use a lysate of whole mycoplasma cells to produce the antigen for the assay.[3,30] This method of antigen preparation is used because it is easily accomplished and yields a reliable, stable antigen for routine use. Several other ELISA antigen preparation methods have been reported[2,45,46,49] and all of these will work satisfactorily, but are not as easy. This general method may be used for all murine mycoplasmas, but the harvesting times and protein yield will vary considerably from species to species. Mycoplasma antigens prepared by this method are stable at −70°C for at least 6 months. The effect of storage conditions on antigenicity must be assessed for each preparation method and for each mycoplasmal species.

1. Harvest (centrifugation at 10,000–20,000 g) 1–3 L of a log phase broth culture of the desired mycoplasma. The pellet may be any shade of white, grey, or even almost black, depending on the species.
2. Wash organisms three times in sterile phosphate buffered saline (PBS) at pH 7.4 by adding PBS at a ratio of ten times the volume of the pellet, mixing well, and then centrifuging the suspension. Pour off the supernatant. Repeat. Resuspend the pellet in a small volume (1–10 ml) of PBS.
3. Transfer a small amount of the final suspension into BHI broth (or other suitable medium) to check for bacterial contamination. Note that *M. pulmonis* will sometimes grow on 5% sheep blood agar plates.
4. Determine protein concentration of the final suspension.
5. Dilute the suspension in sterile PBS to a final concentration of 5 mg protein/ml. Store aliquots of the suspension at −70°C.
6. Dilute a small amount of the 5 mg/ml suspension 1:100 (0.05 ml of suspension to 0.95 ml PBS) and read absorbance at 540 nanometers.
7. Dilute the remainder of the suspension 1:20 in carbonate-bicarbonate buffer (0.05 M, pH 10.0). Incubate the diluted suspension at 37°C.
8. Check the absorbance of the diluted suspension at 5-minute intervals until the absorbance of the suspension is 50% of the absorbance of PBS suspension in step 6. This usually takes about 15 minutes.
9. Stop the lysis by adding 2.2 g of boric acid per 100 ml of suspension.

10. Determine the protein concentration of the lysate. Store aliquots at −70°C.

STANDARDIZATION OF THE ASSAY

In developing an ELISA there are numerous factors that can affect results and their interpretation. The first decision is whether single or multiple dilutions of a test sample will be tested, and whether results will be reported as absorbance, endpoint titration, significant rises in titer, activity as compared to some "standard" serum, or simply positive or negative when compared to a known positive or negative serum sample. At least in the murine system, a single serum sample is adequate for diagnostic purposes. However, single-dilution ELISA assays are heavily dependent on antibody affinity, and therefore, quantitative standardization in terms of milligrams of antibody present is almost impossible.

In setting all dilutions of antibody and reagents, nothing but the amount of antiserum in the unknown test sample should be limiting. Thus, adjusting the concentration of the conjugate or the serum dilution to control nonspecific reactions is likely to cause trouble. Often, these dilutions are set by checkerboard titration of antigen concentration, serum dilution, and conjugate dilution simultaneously, and choosing the conditions that give maximum separation between normal and immune serum. This is likely to lead to conditions in which some factor besides the specific antibody in the test serum is limiting, and also makes replacement of a single reagent difficult and unnecessarily time-consuming. Using the methods described below, one can replace any expended reagents easily, and run only two experiments to determine if the assay is still working correctly.

Selection of solid support

The first step in establishing the assay is choosing an acceptable solid phase support, which is usually a microtiter plate. We obtained two different lot numbers of nine different types of microtiter plates and ran the routine ELISA for IgG[30] with known immune serum to *M. pulmonis* and known negative serum in a repeating pattern so that the variation in results between inside wells, outside wells, and total plate variation could be determined. The experiment was repeated three times on different days. The mean, standard deviation, coefficient of variation, and ratio of immune to normal serum absorbance (405 nm) of the colored product of the alkaline phosphatase reaction was determined for each sample. The coefficient of variation should be as small as possible, and the ratio of the immune to normal serum should be as large as possible. The results are shown in Table 8.4.

We found that all plates showed a significant "edge effect," as has been reported for many serologic tests done in microtiter plates. Therefore, do

Table 8.4. Microtiter plate variation in the mouse IgG ELISA

Plate[a]	Immune Serum Mean(SD)[b]	CoV[b]	Normal Serum Mean(SD)	CoV	Immune/ Normal Ratio[b]
Linbro					
Inside wells	1.69(0.13)	0.08	0.04(0.01)	0.32	39.2
Total	1.73(0.15)	0.09	0.05(0.02)	0.50	35.1
Immulon I					
Inside wells	1.72(0.12)	0.07	0.04(0.02)	0.40	34.1
Total	1.76(0.14)	0.08	0.04(0.02)	0.46	33.9
Falcon Probind					
Inside wells	1.88(0.13)	0.07	0.06(0.04)	0.65	30.5
Total	1.86(0.14)	0.07	0.06(0.04)	0.72	30.1
Immulon II					
Inside wells	1.48(0.11)	0.08	0.04(0.02)	0.34	32.9
Total	1.55(0.15)	0.10	0.71(0.06)	0.82	21.8
Nunc					
Inside wells	1.28(0.16)	0.12	0.05(0.05)	1.05	21.8
Total	1.36(0.20)	0.15	0.10(0.11)	1.08	13.6
Costar-Rigid					
Inside wells	1.24(0.15)	0.12	0.04(0.02)	0.65	31.8
Total	1.30(0.19)	0.14	0.08(0.08)	1.10	17.2
Costar-Flexible					
Inside wells	1.46(0.01)	0.01	0.05(0.01)	0.16	27.7
Total	1.50(0.12)	0.08	0.06(0.04)	1.78	23.2
Corning					
Inside wells	0.42(0.08)	0.18	0.02(0.04)	1.97	20.3
Total	0.51(0.16)	0.30	0.04(0.07)	1.61	11.8
Falcon					
Inside wells	0.31(0.08)	0.25	0.02(0.03)	1.58	17.2
Total	0.37(0.14)	0.37	0.06(0.08)	1.40	6.7

[a]Manufacturer's catalog numbers of plates tested are: Linbro (76–381–04); Immulon I (011–0100–3350); Falcon Probind (3915); Immulon II (011–010–3450); Nunc (439454); Costar-rigid (3590); Costar-flexible (6595); Corning (25860); and Falcon (3072).

[b]Numbers represent the mean (± standard deviation), coefficient of variation (CoV), and ratio between the immune and normal serum for all wells except those on outside edges of the plate (n = 60), or the ratio between immune and normal serum including both the inside and outside wells (n = 90). The CoV should be as small as possible and the ratio of immune to normal serum should be as large as possible. The criteria we feel are acceptable are: CoV less than 0.5–0.75 for both the immune and normal serum, and a large ratio between the immune and normal serum values. Using these criteria, the Linbro, Immulon I, Falcon Probind, and Immulon II plates are acceptable for use in the assay.

not use the outside rows of wells for the test. Also, some plates do not bind the antigen sufficiently to make the test reliable. With such plates, the absorbance readings were much lower than with other plates. The criteria used for selection of a microtiter plate are: coefficient of variation less than 0.5–0.75 for both immune and normal serum, and the highest possible ratio between hyperimmune and normal serum. These values tell one whether or not the values will be reproducible, and the ratio provides the limit to the range of the assay. Obviously, one would like the limits to be as broad as possible, so choose the plate with the highest value for the immune to normal serum ratio. These criteria must be checked for each antigen preparation.

Blocking of unbound sites on the solid phase support

Even after choosing acceptable plates, nonspecific binding is a problem in the assay. In almost all ELISA assays, there remain unbound sites on the microtiter plates that can nonspecifically absorb either immunoglobulin in the sample or conjugated secondary antibody. These unbound sites should be blocked by inert protein so they are no longer available. This decreases the nonspecific background and thus increases the sensitivity of the assay.

We examined the blocking ability of polysorbate, 2% bovine serum albumin (BSA), 5% BSA, 2% fetal calf serum (FCS), and 5% FCS in microtiter plates that had been coated with 2 μg/ml of *M. pulmonis* antigen in each well. Antigen-coated wells were blocked with one of the test solutions and then reacted with either PBS or with normal rat serum followed by conjugated secondary antibody. The results are shown in Figure 8.1. The best blocking was achieved with 2% BSA. The most commonly used blocking agent is polysorbate, which did block the binding of normal serum to some extent, but did not block the binding of the conjugated secondary antibody to the microtiter wells. The choice of blocking reagent to be used must be examined for each microtiter plate and for each antigen preparation.

Dilutions of antigen, test serum, and conjugate

Arbitrarily choose a dilution of the known immune serum and the conjugated secondary antibody that will give a high concentration of these two reagents so that they cannot be the limiting reagents in the assay. We use a 1:32 dilution of immune serum and 1:200 dilution of affinity-purified conjugate. Coat the microtiter plates with various concentrations (0.1–50 μg/ml of protein) of mycoplasma antigen. Run the assay in the routine manner. Plot the absorbance vs. the antigen concentration as shown in Figure 8.2. The absorbance will increase dramatically with the antigen concentration, and reach a plateau after which an increase in antigen concentration will not cause an increase in absorbance. Pick an antigen concentration that is well onto the plateau of the absorbance curve for all future tests. We use a protein concentration of 2 μg/ml, as this ensures that antigen is never the limiting factor in the assay.

The working concentration of each conjugate is determined by reacting antigen-coated wells with PBS, and then using dilutions (1:500–1:10,000) of affinity-purified conjugates in the assay. Plot the absorbance

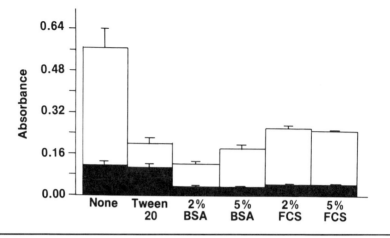

Fig. 8.1. Effect of blocking agents on nonspecific absorption in the ELISA. Microtiter plate wells were coated with 2 μg/ml of *M. pulmonis* antigen and incubated at 37°C overnight with either no blocking agent (PBS), Tween 20, 2% bovine serum albumin in PBS (BSA), 5% BSA, 2% fetal calf serum (FCS) in PBS, or 5% FCS. After incubation, wells were reacted with PBS (closed bars), or with normal rat serum (NRS: open bars). The PBS results indicate the nonspecific absorbance of the conjugate to the wells and antigen. Data were analyzed by analysis of variance. Note that unblocked wells gave an unacceptably high background both with and without serum. Tween 20 blocked the nonspecific absorption of NRS somewhat, but did not affect the nonspecific absorption of the conjugate to the wells. Nonspecific absorption of both normal serum and conjugate was best blocked by incubating antigen-coated plates with 2% BSA.

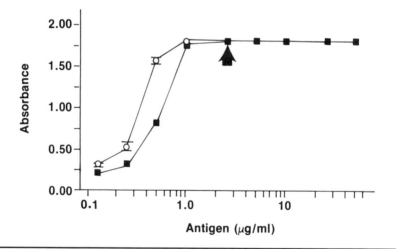

Fig. 8.2. Determination of antigen concentration for the IgG ELISA. Microtiter plates were coated with 0.1–50 μg/ml of *M. pulmonis* protein antigen. Antigen-coated wells were reacted with 1:100 dilution of immune serum followed by 1:500 dilution of the appropriate conjugate. Antigen concentrations greater than 1 μg/ml did not increase absorbance. We use an antigen concentration of 2 μg/ml in the routine assay to ensure that antigen concentration is never the limiting factor in the assay.

vs. the dilution of the conjugate and choose the lowest dilution that does not show appreciable nonspecific binding to the antigen-coated wells as shown in Figure 8.3. As a general rule, the conjugate dilution should be less than 1:5000 to ensure that conjugate is never the limiting factor in the assay. We use a 1:2000 dilution of most affinity-purified conjugates.

The serum dilution to use is the last of these parameters to be determined because one must have already established the working concentrations of antigen and conjugate, and which microtiter plate and blocking reagent works best. The plates are coated with antigen, blocked and reacted with different concentrations of normal rat or mouse serum (dilutions range from 1:10–1:1500), followed by reaction with the conjugate. Plot the absorbance vs. the serum dilution. Choose the lowest dilution that shows little nonspecific absorption to the plates (and therefore, a low absorbance). Sometimes a compromise must be reached at this step (Figure 8.4) because both a very low nonspecific absorbance and a low serum dilution are desirable. The former is necessary for maximum sensitivity, but the latter is required to allow detection of small amounts of antibody. We use a 1:200 dilution of serum.

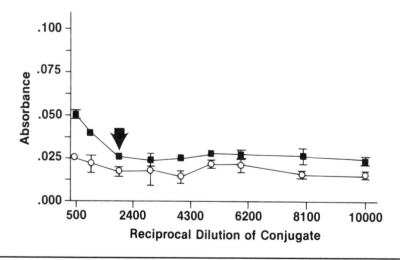

Fig. 8.3. Determination of conjugate dilution for ELISA. *M. pulmonis* antigen-coated wells (2 μg/ml protein) were blocked with 2% BSA followed by incubation with dilutions of affinity purified conjugate. Data for the rat IgG conjugate (squares) are shown. The circles represent the absorbance values from control wells in which the *M. pulmonis* antigen was omitted. These wells measure the amount of nonspecific binding of the conjugate to the plastic. The lowest dilution (1:2000; arrow) of conjugate that did not have appreciable nonspecific binding to the antigen was chosen as the conjugate concentration for the ELISA.

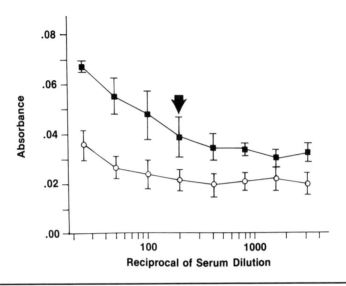

Fig. 8.4. Determination of serum concentration for ELISA. *M. pulmonis* antigen-coated wells (2 μg/ml protein) were blocked with 2% BSA and reacted with dilutions of normal rat (squares) or mouse (circles) serum followed by incubation with 1:2000 dilution of the appropriate IgG conjugate. In choosing the serum dilution to use, a compromise must be reached between the minimum nonspecific absorption of the conjugate (1:400 dilution) and the ability to detect low concentrations of antibody present in the serum. We chose a 1:200 dilution (arrow) of serum for both the rat and mouse ELISAs because the absorbance obtained with this dilution was not significantly different from that obtained with a 1:400 dilution for either serum, but did have significantly less nonspecific absorption of the conjugate than did a 1:50 serum dilution. Data were analyzed by analysis of variance and Duncan's multiple range test.

As a final check of the reaction reagents, the conjugate titration should be run again with normal and immune sera as well as the PBS control. When the absorbance is plotted vs. the conjugate dilution, the normal serum and PBS control curves should be virtually identical, and there should be a wide separation between the values of the immune serum and the normal serum at the conjugate dilution previously selected for use in the assay (Figure 8.5). For example, at the concentrations used for the routine IgG *M. pulmonis* ELISA, we obtain absorbance values of approximately 0.01 for the normal serum and PBS controls, and approximately 1.0 for the immune serum.

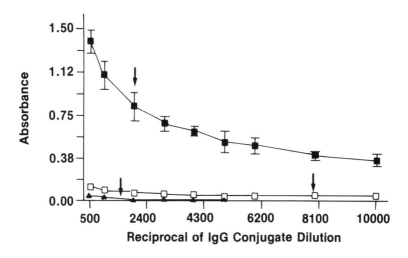

Fig. 8.5. Differential between immune serum and controls. Data for the rat IgG ELISA are shown. Microtiter plate wells were coated with 2 μg/ml of *M. pulmonis* antigen and blocked with 2% BSA. Wells were then reacted with a 1:100 dilution of either normal serum (open squares), immune serum (closed squares), or 2% PBS (triangles). Dilutions of the conjugate were added and absorbance of samples determined. The 1:2000 dilution of the conjugate (arrow) allows adequate separation between the absorbance values for the immune serum and the normal serum. Note that the absorbance values for the 2% BSA negative control and the normal serum are similar. Similar curves were obtained for the mouse IgG and rat and mouse IgM ELISAs.

Incubation times

A wide variety of incubation conditions have been reported for ELISAs. The conditions for each incubation step are determined by methods similar to those used to determine which microtiter plates are acceptable. Mouse and rat immune and normal serum and PBS are run in the assay with the reagents set as determined above. The incubations at each step are varied, one at a time, to determine the effect on the results. The mean, standard deviation, coefficient of variation, and ratio of the absorbance of the immune to normal serum are determined for each incubation procedure. An example of determining conjugate incubation conditions is shown in Table 8.5. Once again, the coefficient of variation should be as small as possible, indicating reproducibility, and the ratio of immune to normal serum absorbance values should be as large as possible, indicating the range of the assay and its potential sensitivity. In addition, determine the ratio of

Table 8.5.   Effects of conjugate incubation times

	Incubation Conditions					
	25°C, 3 Hours		25°C, 19.5 Hours		4°C, 19.5 Hours	
Sample[a]	Mean(SD)[b]	CoV[b]	Mean(SD)	CoV	Mean(SD)	CoV
Rat Immune	0.76(0.27)	0.36	1.54(0.04)	0.03	1.29(0.21)	0.16
2% BSA	0.04(0.0)	0.10	0.03(0.0)	0.13	0.03(0.0)	0.13
Rat normal	0.04(0.0)	0.10	0.04(0.0)	0.10	0.03(0.0)	0.13
Immune/normal ratio[c]		19.0		38.5		43.0
Normal/2% BSA ratio[d]		1.0		1.3		1.0
Mouse immune	0.43(0.05)	0.12	1.04(0.04)	0.03	0.89(0.04)	0.04
2% BSA	0.03(0.0)	0.13	0.02(0.0)	0.15	0.02(0.0)	0.15
Mouse normal	0.03(0.0)	0.13	0.02(0.0)	0.15	0.02(0.0)	0.15
Immune/normal ratio[c]		14.3		52.0		44.5
Normal/2% BSA ratio[d]		1.0		1.0		1.0

Note: Goat anti-rat IgG and goat anti-mouse IgG were used at a 1:2000 dilution in phosphate buffered saline (PBS) at pH 7.4.)

[a] Rat and mouse immune sera were used at a 1:1024 dilution in PBS. Normal rat and mouse sera were used at a 1:200 dilution in PBS. BSA is a 2% solution (w/v) of bovine serum albumin in PBS. This solution is used to block nonspecific binding of the conjugate in the assay. Therefore, this sample serves as a negative control for the assay.

[b] Numbers represent the mean (± standard deviation) and coefficient of variation (CoV) for 20 values for each test sample, run on two separate days. The CoV should be as small as possible.

[c] Value is the mean of the values for the immune serum divided by the mean of the values for the normal serum. Value should be as large as possible.

[d] Value is the mean of the values for the normal serum divided by the mean of the values for the 2% BSA negative control. This ratio represents activity due to nonspecific binding of the conjugate. This value should be as close to 1 as possible.

the normal serum to the PBS control values because this is a measure of the nonspecific activity in the system. This ratio should be as close to 1 as possible, thereby indicating no nonspecific activity.

QUALITY CONTROL OF THE ASSAY

One of the disadvantages of the ELISA assay is its extreme sensitivity to changes in procedure. If a minor variation is inadvertently introduced into the procedure at one point, this variation may be amplified by the test. Therefore, stringent quality control measures are required. We have found the Youden plot[32] to be very useful. This method requires the use of dilutions of immune serum simulating high, midrange, and low concentrations of specific antibody to the antigen in question (Figure 8.6). To determine within-run and between-run variability in the assay, one sample of each dilution is run at the beginning of a set of samples, and another is included at the end of the assay. The absorbance values obtained on these control samples are plotted against each other, resulting in a linear plot with a slope of 1 at a 45° angle from the X and Y axis (Figure 8.7). Variability within an assay is indicated by the spread of points away from the 45° line. The maximum divergence from the line should be no more than 10% deviation.

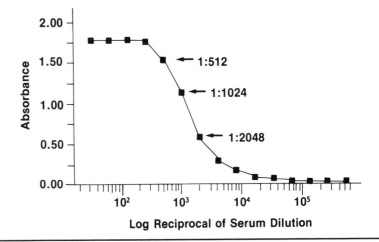

Fig. 8.6. Choice of serum samples for quality control of ELISA. Data for the rat IgG ELISA are shown. Microtiter plate wells were coated with 2 μg/ml of *M. pulmonis* antigen, blocked with 2% BSA, reacted with dilutions of the immune serum and a 1:2000 dilution of the conjugate. Dilutions of 1:512, 1:1024, and 1:2048 (arrows) were chosen as the high, medium, and low antibody concentrations for quality control samples because they are on the linear part of the dilution curve. Similar curves were obtained for the other assays.

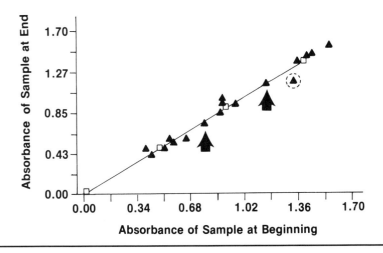

Fig. 8.7. Use of the Youden plot for quality control of ELISA. Data for one month of the mouse IgG assay are shown. Points (open squares) on the 45° line indicate the means of the last month's absorbance values for the 2% BSA-negative control, and the high (1:512 dilution of immune serum), medium (1:1024 dilution of immune serum), and low (1:2048 dilution of immune serum) concentrations of anti-*M. pulmonis* antibody. Points for individual test runs are indicated by triangles. The arrows indicate assays that were unacceptable because both the high and medium control sera deviated by more than 10% from the mean values obtained in the previous month. Note that there was minimal intra-assay variation (i.e., variation away from the 45° line). The greatest deviation (indicated by broken circle) was within a 10% deviation for both within-assay and between-assay variation.

Day-to-day variation is indicated by the spread of values away from the averages of the last 10 assay runs. If a value for an individual day deviates by more than 10% from the average of the values for the last 10 runs, the run should be repeated. Other indications that a run needs to be repeated are that all three samples fall on one side of the line and are outside of a 5% deviation range.

LIMITATIONS

The ELISA has many advantages, but depends on the ability of the animal to produce specific antibody. In very young or very old animals, and in T and B cell-deficient rodents, antibody production may be minimal or completely lacking. Also, a delay in production of antibody to subclinical infections results in a 1–3 month "lag time" when infected animals cannot be detected by serologic methods.[4] Since this usually occurs after the time of weaning, when most rodents are purchased and used, it is generally impossible for the user to detect infected animals upon their arrival. Detection of early infection and infection due to small numbers of organisms can be improved by detective specific anti-*M. pulmonis* IgM. Following experimental inoculation of specific pathogen-free rats with 10^1 CFU of *M. pulmonis,* the IgM ELISA detects 17% of exposed animals as compared to 7% for the IgG assay. Comparable figures for inoculation with 10^3 CFU are 24% vs. 13%.[18]

Unfortunately, major problems remain with the use of the ELISA as a diagnostic method for murine mycoplasmas. The quality control procedures to ensure reliable results are rigorous, but most challenging are the cross-reactions among the murine mycoplasmas.[4,6,21,60] All of the murine mycoplasmas share some common antigens; these appear to be particularly troublesome in trying to discriminate *M. pulmonis* infection from *M. arthritidis* or *M. muris* infection.[4,6,60]

Several methods have been attempted to improve the species specificity of the mycoplasma ELISA. These include the development of an *M. arthritidis* ELISA, use of immunoblots to verify ELISA results, blocking of cross-reactive antibodies with rabbit antisera, precipitation of cross-reactive antibodies with heterologous organisms, and removal of cross-reactive antigens by affinity chromatography.[3,4,6,11,21,60] The ELISA for *M. arthritidis* has never been field-tested or even extensively tested with experimental infections. In low-dose experimental infections, the cross-reactions between *M. pulmonis* and *M. arthritidis* are sufficiently strong that there are minimal differences between the magnitude of the responses to the homologous or heterologous organisms.[8,16] Furthermore, there is little hope that this method can ever be useful in recognizing animals infected with both organisms. All of the methods to improve species specificity have proven difficult to standardize, especially removal by affinity chromatography, as there is no way to monitor whether remaining activity is still cross-reactive or specific. Finally, with the exception of immunoblots, these stopgap measures are not helpful in the diagnosis of mixed infections.

Immunoblots

Immunoblots have been widely used as specific tests to identify a large number of infections, including AIDS.[12] We use the one-dimensional SDS polyacrylamide gel electrophoresis (SDS-PAGE) method of Laemmli[34] to separate mycoplasma proteins, and the method of Towbin, Staehelin, and Gordon[59] to transfer the proteins to nitrocellulose sheets. Mycoplasma proteins are identified by reacting the blotted proteins with sera from mice or rats suspected to be infected with mycoplasmas.

Normally, we use immunoblots only to achieve a specific diagnosis when ELISA results indicate that a given colony is infected with one of the murine mycoplasmas. In addition to a battery of test sera from the colony and protein preparations of all murine mycoplasmal species, positive and negative controls are required: immune sera from experimentally infected mice or rats and normal sera from animals known to be mycoplasma-free, respectively. The preparation of mycoplasma proteins for electrophoresis is as follows:

SDS EXTRACT OF MYCOPLASMAS

1. Grow mycoplasmas to late log phase of growth cycle in appropriate medium. Harvest mycoplasmas by centrifugation, and wash cells three times with sterile 0.85% NaCl or PBS. Resuspend pellet in sterile 0.85% NaCl or PBS. Suspension should be cloudy.
2. Determine protein concentration of suspension. Freeze ($-70°C$) 200-μg aliquots until needed. Storage in screw-cap microfuge tubes is convenient.
3. Centrifuge cells at approximately 14,000 g. Discard the supernatant.
4. Add 1 μl of dissociation buffer (see below) for each μg protein (i.e., 200 μl). Resuspend pellet. Replace screw cap. Drill a small hole in the top (to allow the steam to escape in step 5). A hot wire, needle, or straightened paper clip works nicely as a drill.
5. Boil sample for 2–4 minutes in a water bath. Sample must be tightly capped to prevent evaporation.
6. Add 100 μl (for 200 μg protein) of lysis buffer (see below). The final concentration of protein is 1 μg/μl.
7. Freeze sample. For short-term storage, $-20°C$ is fine, but $-70°C$ is recommended for long-term storage.
8. Before using the sample, centrifuge it in a microfuge (14,000 g). Do

not use any of the pelleted material because it is not solubilized.
9. Normal loading of gels is 20 μg protein per well.

Dissociation buffer without 2-mercaptoethanol

1 M Tris buffer, pH 6.8	31.25	ml
SDS	1.5	gm
Glycerol (glycerin)*	50	gm*
Ultrapure water, QS to 500 ml		

Filter solution through a 0.2-μm filter.

*Weigh glycerol and rinse weighing container with ultrapure water. This solution can be stored at room temperature.

Lysis buffer

Urea	11.4	gm
10% NP40*	4	ml
Mercaptoethanol (2-ME)	1	ml
Ampholines, pH 5–7	0.8	ml
Ampholines, pH 3–10	0.2	ml
Ultrapure water	5.32	ml

*10 ml of Nonidet-P40 (Sigma Chemical Company, St. Louis, MO) in 100 ml of ultrapure water. This solution must be stored at −20°C.

LIMITATIONS

While immunoblots are relatively expensive, time-consuming, technically complicated, and impractical for screening large numbers of samples, they are the preferred method for achieving a specific diagnosis in a barrier-maintained colony in which there are a few ELISA-positive animals. The approach is based on the assumption that sera from infected animals should recognize more protein antigens from the infecting organism than from any of the other murine mycoplasmas. If the pattern of bands is sufficiently complex (i.e., 10 or more bands are present), it is relatively easy to make a specific diagnosis.[4,16,21] Furthermore, dual infections can be recognized by the presence of a complex banding pattern to more than one organism. However, in about 50% of cases, less than 4 bands are seen with any antigen, or only bands known to be cross-reacting proteins are present.[16,21] Based on results from long-term monitoring of a barrier-maintained colony, the pattern seen with any single animal's serum often begins as 1–4 bands, and complete patterns develop only after the animal has been infected for several months.[16] Thus, months of repeat-testing of the same animals may be required before a definite diagnosis can be made.

Recommendations

At the present time, there is no fully satisfactory diagnostic test for the murine mycoplasmas that is applicable to all situations. The combination of diagnostic tests chosen must be adapted to the desired goal and the results must be interpreted with caution. The easiest situation in which to make a diagnosis is a conventional colony. Virtually all conventional rodent colonies are infected with *M. pulmonis,* and these infections are easily detected by several methods. Agreement between cultural and ELISA results in these colonies is approximately 98%. It is much more difficult to develop a screening program for barrier-maintained rats and mice housed in a well managed colony that contains no agents known to exacerbate mycoplasmal infections and in which most of the animals are used at weaning. In this case, if a mycoplasma is present, only a small number of the animals may be actually infected, and those that are infected will have few organisms. The ELISA should be the test of choice for initial screening barrier-maintained colonies of laboratory rodents for mycoplasma infection. Breeding colonies should be monitored monthly by including as many animals of all subpopulations (i.e., room, rack, strain, etc.) as possible. Breeding animals, preferably retired breeders at least 6 months old, should be tested by both the IgG and IgM ELISA for *M. pulmonis*. Weanling animals are generally ELISA-negative.[4,16,21] If positive animals are found, one must decide whether or not to exclude all mycoplasmas or just *M. pulmonis*. If one decides to exclude *M. pulmonis* only, then some discriminatory test is necessary to determine whether or not this organism is present. Multiple site sampling for culture of both *M. pulmonis* and *M. arthritidis* (the two most commonly isolated species) and immunoblots of the serum against all of the murine mycoplasma species are possible verification methods. Neither of these methods works in all instances, but use of the ELISA backed up by culture and immunoblots gives about an 80% chance of identifying *M. pulmonis* if it is present. If neither *M. pulmonis* nor *M. arthritidis* is identified in the colony, one should continue to retest animals from the colony monthly until definite evidence for the mycoplasmal species involved is obtained.

If one decides that no mycoplasmas are desired in the colony, one may have an additional problem. Three mycoplasmal species, *M. pulmonis, M. arthritidis,* and *M. muris,* have been isolated from the genital tract. Therefore, cesarian derivation to eliminate the organisms may be difficult or impossible. Finding mycoplasma-free foster mothers for the animals may also be difficult. A possible approach, which unfortunately has not been tested, would be to give several pregnant females Ciprofloxacin (Miles, Inc., West Haven, CT) during pregnancy, cesarian-derive the pups, house each litter in a separate Trexler plastic film isolator, and hand rear the pups. Even then, each stock would have to be monitored monthly for at least a year before one would know if the attempt was successful.

If a colony is ELISA-negative on the initial screening and remains so for several months, the sensitivity of the ELISA to detect a new infection with *M. pulmonis* can be improved by using the negative serum from the colony as the negative internal standard for the assay. Use of such control serum and the IgM ELISA more than doubles the chance of detecting infection within the first 28 days following experimental infection with less than 10^6 CFU of *M. pulmonis.*[18]

There simply is no way with current methods to prove, by a single test or a battery of tests, that a given population of weanling mice or rats is mycoplasma-free. Barrier-maintained weanling animals between 2 and 4 months old are generally culturally and ELISA-negative.[4,16,21] Thus, it is impossible to verify that weanling animals obtained from commercial breeders are free of *M. pulmonis.* One option is to obtain the dams of the animals one wants to use, and do multiple site culturing and ELISA-testing on the dams. Obviously, an assay sensitive enough to detect infection with *M. pulmonis,* or any of the other murine mycoplasmas in weanling animals, needs to be developed. Two possibilities that seem feasible with current technology are the development of specific mycoplasmal antigen detection assays or DNA hybridization methods using specific gene probes with the polymerase chain reaction.[50] Unfortunately, it will probably require at least 2–5 years for such assays to be developed and adequately field-tested.

References

1. Broderson JR, Lindsey JR, Crawford JE: 1976, The role of environmental ammonia in respiratory mycoplasmosis of rats. Am J Pathol 85: 115–30.

2. Bruggman S, Keller H: 1977, Quantitative detection of antibodies to *Mycoplasma suipneumoniae* in pig's sera by an enzyme-linked immunosorbent assay. Vet Rec 101: 109–111.

3. Cassell GH, Brown MB: 1983, Enzyme-linked immunosorbent assay (ELISA) for detection of anti-mycoplasmal antibody. In: Methods in mycoplasmology, eds. Razin S, Tully JG, Vol. I, pp. 457–469. Academic Press, New York, NY.

4. Cassell GH, Cox NR, Davis JK, Brown MB, Minion FC, Lindsey JR: 1986, State of the art detection methods for rodent mycoplasmas. In: Complications of viral and mycoplasmal infections in rodents to toxicology research and testing, ed. Hamm Jr TE, pp.143–160. Hemisphere Press, Washington, DC.

5. Cassell G H, Davidson MK, Davis JK, Lindsey JR: 1983, Recovery and identification of murine mycoplasmas. In: Methods in mycoplasmology, eds. Razin S, Tully JG, Vol. II, pp. 129–142. Academic Press, New York, NY.

6. Cassell GH, Davis JK, Cox NR, Davidson MK, Lindsey JR: 1984, *Mycoplasma pulmonis* detection in rodents: Lessons for diagnosis in other species. Isr J Med Sci 20: 859–865.

7. Cassell G H, Davis JK, Lindsey JR, Davidson MK, Brown MB, Baker HJ: 1983, Detection of *Mycoplasma pulmonis* infections by ELISA. Lab Animal 12: 27–38.

8. Cassell G H, Davis JK, Simecka JW, Lindsey JR, Cox NR, Ross S, Fallon M: 1986, Mycoplasmal infections: Disease pathogenesis, implications for biomedical research, and control. In: Viral and mycoplasmal infections of laboratory rodents, eds. Bhatt PN, Murphy FA, pp. 87–129. Academic Press, New York, NY.

9. Cassell GH, Hill A: 1979, Murine and other small animal mycoplasmas. In: The mycoplasmas, eds. Tully JG, Whitcomb RF, Vol, II, pp. 235–273. Academic Press, New York, NY.

10. Cassell GH, Lindsey JR, Baker HJ, Davis JK: 1979, Mycoplasmal and rickettsial diseases. In: The laboratory rat, eds. Baker HJ, Lindsey JR, Weisbroth SH, Vol. I, pp. 243–269. Academic Press, New York, NY.

11. Cassell GH, Lindsey JR, Davis JK, Davidson MK, Brown MB, Mayo JA: 1981, Detection of *Mycoplasma pulmonis* infection in rats and mice by an enzyme-linked immunosorbent assay (ELISA). Lab Anim Sci 31: 676–682.

12. United States Department of Health and Human Services, Public Health Services, Centers for Disease Control, Center for Infectious Diseases, AIDS Program: 1989, Interpretation and Use of the Western Blot Assay for Serodiagnosis of Human Immunodeficiency Virus Type 1 Infections. Morbidity and Mortality Weekly Report 38: Supplement 7.

13. Clyde W A: 1983, Growth inhibition tests. In: Methods in mycoplasmology, eds. Razin S, Tully JG, Vol. I, pp. 405–410. Academic Press, New York, NY.

14. Cole BC, Miller ML, Ward JR: 1969, The role of mycoplasma arthritis induced by 6-sulfanilamidoindazole (6-SAI). Proc Soc Exp Biol Med 130: 994–1000.

15. Committee on long-term holding of laboratory rodents: 1976, Long-term holding of laboratory rodents. ILAR News 19: L1–L25.

16. Cox NR, Davidson MK, Davis JK, Lindsey JR, Cassell GH: 1988, Natural mycoplasmal infections in isolator-maintained LEW/Tru rats. Lab Anim Sci 38: 381–388.

17. Davidson MK, Lindsey JR, Brown MB, Cassell GH, Boorman G: 1983, Natural infection of *Mycoplasma arthritidis* in mice. Curr Microbiol 8: 205–208.

18. Davidson MK, Lindsey JR, Brown MB, Schoeb TR, Cassell GH: 1981, Comparison of methods for detection of *Mycoplasma pulmonis* in experimentally and naturally infected rats. J Clin Microbiol 14:646–655.

19. Davidson MK, Lindsey JR, Parker RF, Tully JG, Cassell GH: 1988, Differences in virulence for mice among strains of *Mycoplasma pulmonis*. Infect Immun 56: 2156–2162.

20. Davis JK, Cassell GH: 1982, Murine respiratory mycoplasmosis in LEW and F344 rats: Strain differences in lesion severity. Vet Pathol 19: 280–293.

21. Davis JK, Cassell GH, Gambill G, Cox N, Watson H, Davidson M: 1986, Diagnosis of murine mycoplasmal infections by enzyme-linked immunosorbent assay (ELISA). Isr J Med Sci 23: 717–722.

22. Davis JK, Parker RF, White H, Dziedzic D, Taylor G, Davidson MK, Cox NR, Cassell GH: 1985, Strain differences in susceptibility to murine respiratory mycoplasmosis in C57BL/6 and C3H/HeN mice. Infect Immun 50: 647–654.

23. Freundt EA: 1983, Principles of mycoplasma classification and taxonomy. In: Methods in mycoplasmology, eds. Razin S, Tully JG, Vol. I, pp. 9–14. Academic Press, New York, NY.

24. Freundt EA: 1983, Culture media for classic mycoplasmas. In: Methods in mycoplasmology, eds. Razin S, Tully JG, Vol. I, pp. 127–146. Academic Press, New York, NY.

25. Ganaway JR, Spencer TH, Moore TD, Allen AM: 1985, Isolation, propagation, and characterization of a newly recognized pathogen, cilia-associated respiratory bacillus of rats, an etiological agent of chronic respiratory disease. Infect Immun 47: 472–479.

26. Gardella RS, DelGiudice RA, Tully JG: 1983, Immunofluorescence. In: Methods in mycoplasmology, eds. Razin S, Tully JG, Vol. I, pp. 431–440. Academic Press, New York, NY.

27. Giebel J, Binder A, Koh HB, Kirchhoff H: 1988, Isolation of mycoplasmas from

intestine of rat, swine, and man. Abstracts of the Seventh International Congress of the International Organization for Mycoplasmology, Baden near Vienna, Austria.

28. Hill A: 1978, Demonstration of mycoplasmas in tissues by the immunoperoxidase technique. J Infect Dis 137: 152–154.

29. Hill AC: 1983, *Mycoplasma collis,* a new species from rats and mice. Internat J Syst Bacteriol 33: 847–851.

30. Horowitz SA, Cassell GH: 1978, Detection of antibodies to *Mycoplasma pulmonis* by an enzyme-linked immunosorbent assay. Infect Immun 22:161–170.

31. International Committee on Systematic Bacteriology, Subcommittee on the Taxonomy of *Mollicutes:* 1979, Proposal of minimal standards for descriptions of new species of the class *Mollicutes.* Internat J Sys Bacteriol 29: 172–180.

32. Jeffcoate SL: 1982, Use of Youden plot for internal quality control on the immunoassay laboratory. Ann Clin Biochem. 19:435–437.

33. Kirchhoff H: Institut für Mikrobiologie und Tierseuchen Tierärztlichen Hochschule Hannover. Hannover, Germany, Personal communication.

34. Laemmli UK: 1970, Cleavage of structural proteins during assembly of bacteriophage T4. Nature 227: 680–685.

35. Lang CM (Chairman): 1980, National Survey of Laboratory Animal Facilities and Resources, Fiscal Year 1978. Institute of Laboratory Animal Resources, National Academy of Sciences. NIH Pub No 80-2091. USDHHS, NIH, Bethesda, MD.

36. Lindsey JR: 1986, Prevalence of viral and mycoplasmal infections in laboratory rodents. In: Viral and mycoplasmal infections of laboratory rodents: Effects on biomedical research, eds. Bhatt PN, Jacoby RO, Morse HC, New AE, pp. 801–808. Academic Press, New York, NY.

37. Lindsey JR, Baker HJ, Overcash RG, Cassell GH, Hunt CE: 1971, Murine chronic respiratory disease. Significance as a research complication and experimental production with *Mycoplasma pulmonis.* Am J Pathol 64: 675–716.

38. Lindsey JR, Casebolt DB, Cassell GH: 1986, Animal health in toxicological research: An appraisal of past performance and future prospects. In: Managing conduct and data quality of toxicology studies, pp. 155–171. Princeton Scientific Press, Princeton, NJ.

39. Lindsey JR, Cassell GH, Baker HJ: 1978, Diseases due to mycoplasmas and rickettsias. In: Pathology of laboratory animals, eds. Benirschke K, Garner FM, Jones TC, pp. 1481–1550. Springer-Verlag, New York, NY.

40. Lindsey JR, Cassell GH, Davidson MK: 1982, Mycoplasmal and other bacterial diseases of the respiratory system. In: The mouse in biomedical research, eds. Foster HL, Small JD, Fox JG, Vol. II, pp. 21–41. Academic Press. New York, NY.

41. Lindsey JR, Davidson MK, Schoeb TR, Cassell GH: 1986, Murine mycoplasmal infections. In: Complications of viral and mycoplasmal infections in rodents to toxicology research and testing, ed. Hamm, Jr TE, pp. 91–121, Hemisphere Press, Washington, DC.

42. Lutsky I, Livni N, Mor N: 1986, Retrospective confirmation of mycoplasma infection by the immunoperoxidase technique. Pathol 18: 390–392.

43. McGarrity GH, Rose DL, Kwiatkowski V, Dion AS, Phillips DM, Tully JG: 1983, *Mycoplasma muris,* a new species from laboratory mice. Internat J Syst Bacteriol 33:350–355.

44. Nelson JB: 1950, Association of a special strain of pleuropneumonia-like organisms with conjunctivitis in a mouse colony. J Exp Med 91: 309–320.

45. Nicolet J, Paroz P, Bruggman S: 1980, Tween 20 soluble proteins of *Mycoplasma hyopneumoniae* as antigen for an enzyme-linked immunosorbent assay. Res Vet Sci 79: 305–309.

46. Onoviran O, Taylor-Robinson D: 1979, Detection of antibody against *Mycoplasma mycoides* sub. *mycoides* in cattle by enzyme-linked immunosorbent assay. Vet Rec 105: 165–167.

47. Parker RF, Davis JK, Cassell GH, White H, Dziedzic D, Blalock DK, Thorp RB, Simecka JW: 1989, Short-term exposure to nitrogen dioxide enhances susceptibility to murine respiratory mycoplasmosis and decreases intrapulmonary killing of *Mycoplasma pulmonis*. Am Rev Resp Dis 140: 502–512.

48. Polak-Vogelzang AA, Hagenaars R, Nagel J: 1978, Evaluation of an immunoperoxidase test for identification of acholeplasma and mycoplasma. J Gen Microbiol 106: 241–249.

49. Raisanen SM, Suni J, Leinikki P: 1980, Serological diagnosis of *Mycoplasma pneumoniae* infection by enzyme assay. J Clin Pathol 33: 836–840.

50. Saiki RK, Gelfand DH, Stoffel S, Scharf SJ, Higuchi R, Horn GJ, Mullis KB, Erlich HA: 1988, Primer-detected enzymatic amplification of DNA with a thermostable DNA polymerase. Science 239:487–491.

51. Sainte-Marie G: 1962, A paraffin embedding technique for studies employing immunofluorescence. J Histochem Cytochem 10: 250–256.

52. Saito M, Nakagawa M, Suzuki E: 1981, Synergistic effect of Sendai virus on *Mycoplasma pulmonis* infection in mice. Jpn J Vet Sci 43: 43–50.

53. Saito M, Nakayama K, Muto T, Nakagawa M: 1982, Effects of gaseous ammonia on *Mycoplasma pulmonis* infection in rats and mice. Exp Animal 31: 203–206.

54. Schoeb TR, Davidson MK, Lindsey JR: 1982, Intracage ammonia promotes growth of *Mycoplasma pulmonis* in the respiratory tract of rats. Infect Immun 38: 212–217.

55. Schoeb TR, Kervin KC, Lindsey JR: 1985, Exacerbation of murine respiratory mycoplasmosis in gnotobiotic F344/N rats by Sendai virus infection. Vet Pathol 22: 272–282.

56. Schoeb TR, Lindsey JR: 1987, Exacerbation of murine respiratory mycoplasmosis by sialodacryoadenitis virus in gnotobiotic F344 rats. Vet Pathol 24: 392–399.

57. Schreiber H, Nettesheim P, Linjinsky W, Richter CB, Walburg HE Jr: 1972, Induction of lung cancer in germ free, specific pathogen free and infected rats by N-nitroso-hepatamethyleneimine: enhancement of respiratory infection. J Natl Cancer Inst 4:1107–1114.

58. Taylor-Robinson D, Chen TA: 1983, Growth inhibitory factors in animal and plant tissues. In: Methods in mycoplasmology, eds. Razin S, Tully JG, Vol. I, pp. 109–114. Academic Press, New York, NY.

59. Towbin H, Staehelin T, Gordon J: 1979, Electrophoretic transfer of proteins from polyacrylamide gels to nitrocellulose sheets: Procedure and some applications. Proc Natl Acad Sci USA. 76: 4350–4354.

60. Watson HL, Cox NR, Davidson MK, Blalock DK, Davis JK, Dybvig K, Horowitz SA, Cassell GH: 1987, *Mycoplasma pulmonis* proteins common to the murine mycoplasmas. Isr J Med Sci 23: 442–447.

61. Whitcomb RF: 1983, Culture media for spiroplasmas. In: Methods in mycoplasmology, eds. Razin S, Tully JG, Vol. I, pp. 147–162. Academic Press, New York, NY.

APPENDIX A8.1.   Media Formulations for Murine Mycoplasmas

Medium A for Murine Mycoplasmas

MATERIALS

Mycoplasma broth base (Frey, BBL Microbiology Systems, Cockeysville, MD)

SeaPlaque agarose or Noble agar (Difco Laboratories, Detroit, MI)

DNA (degraded free acid type IV, Sigma Chemical, St. Louis, MO)

Agamma horse serum, heat inactivated for 30 minutes at 56°C (GG Free Horse Serum, GIBCO/BRL, Grand Island, NY)

Dextrose, aqueous, 50% (w/v) solution (Sigma, 50 g anhydrous dextrose/100 ml ultrapure water, filter-sterilized)

L-arginine HCl, aqueous, 42% (w/v) solution (Difco, 42 g/100ml ultrapure water, filter-sterilized)

Phenol red, 1% (w/v) solution in methanol or isopropanol (Fisher Chemicals, West Haven, CT)

Cefobid, cefoperazone sodium, 250 mg/ml stock solution of IV- or IM-injectable drug (Roerig/Pfizer, New York, NY)

Ultrapure water, 18 ohm, reagent grade, preferably endotoxin-free, or tissue culture-quality double-distilled water

NaOH, concentrated solution in ultrapure water to adjust pH

NaOH, 1N solution in ultrapure water for minor pH adjustments

HCl, 1N solution in ultrapure water for minor pH adjustments

Petri dishes, sterile, irradiated – not gas sterilized, for agar plates

Sterile tubes or bottles for dispensing broth

Autoclave

Water bath, 55°C, for agar only

0.22 μm sterile filtration units

pH meter and calibration buffers

Stir bars and stir plate

Graduated cylinder, sterile, for adding large amounts of serum

PREPARATION

For 200 ml of medium (see discussion below before proceeding):

1. Add these ingredients to ultrapure, endotoxin-free water and mix well.

Mycoplasma broth base	4.5	g
DNA	0.04	g
Ultrapure water	157	ml
Phenol red (indicator, optional)	0.4	ml
FOR AGAR MEDIUM ONLY		
Agar (SeaPlaque or Noble)	2	g

2. After ingredients are mixed, use concentrated NaOH to adjust pH to 7.8–8.0 for glucose utilizers (*M. pulmonis, M. neurolyticum, M. collis*). Use 1 N HCl to adjust pH to 7.0 for arginine utilizer (*M. arthritidis*).
3. Autoclave medium at 121°C with 15 pounds pressure (slow exhaust or liquids cycle) for 15 minutes. Allow medium to cool. Medium

containing agar should be placed in a 55°C water bath to prevent solidification.

4. Aseptically add:

Agamma horse serum	40 ml
50% dextrose	2 ml
OR	
42% arginine	1 ml

NOTE: Both glucose and arginine can be incorporated into the same medium, but arginine can inhibit the growth of some glucose utilizers.

5. Antimicrobial agents;

Cefobid	52 μl

NOTE: The half-life of Cefobid in broth or agar is about 7 days at 2–8°C. Therefore, add more penicillin to broth after it has been stored so the concentration of the antimicrobial is high enough to inhibit bacterial growth. If agar plates are to be stored more than 1 week, add twice the amount of Cefobid to the medium so there will be enough antibiotic left after 1 week to inhibit bacterial growth. This concentration of Cefobid is safe for mycoplasmas.

6. Store broth and agar at 2–8°C. Broth will remain stable for 1 month at this temperature. Broth may be frozen (-20°C) for 3 months. If there is a precipitate in the medium after freezing, discard the precipitate. (This phenomenon varies among lots of horse serum.)

7. Aseptically dispense broth as needed into sterile petri dishes. Sea-Plaque agarose is a low-gelling-temperature agarose so agar plates will take longer than usual to solidify at 22–25°C. Agar will not solidify at warmer room temperatures.

DISCUSSION

1. Use the manufacturer's instructions for the amount of base (usually given in grams per liter). This amount may vary slightly from lot to lot.

2. Agar preparations can stratify. Be sure the serum and solutions added after autoclaving are well mixed before dispensing final medium. An easy method of mixing is to include a stir bar in the medium before autoclaving, then mix the final medium well, on a stir plate, before dispensing. If the room is very cool, it may be necessary to keep the agar in a 50°C water bath or on a heated stir plate while dispensing.

References

1. Cassell GH, Davidson MK, Davis JK, Lindsey JR: 1983, Recovery and identification of murine mycoplasmas, In: Methods in Mycoplasmology, eds. Tully JG, Razin S, Vol II., pp 129–142. Academic Press, New York, NY.

2. Davidson MK, Lindsey JR, Brown MB, 1983. Natural *Mycoplasma arthritidis* infection in mice. Curr Microbiol 8: 205–208.

3. Davidson MK, Lindsey JR, Parker RF, Tully JG, Cassell GH: 1988, Differences in virulence for mice among strains of *Mycoplasma pulmonis*. Infect Immun 56: 2156–2162.

SP4 Medium for *Mycoplasma muris*

MATERIALS

Mycoplasma broth base w/o crystal violet (BBL)
SeaPlaque agarose (FMC—preferred) or Noble agar (Difco)
Bacto-peptone (Difco)
Bacto-tryptone (Difco)
Yeastolate (Difco), 2% aqueous solution
Dextrose (Sigma)
CMRL-1066 tissue culture medium with glutamine; 10× solution (GIBCO/BRL)
Fetal bovine serum, heat-inactivated for 30 minutes at 56°C (GIBCO/BRL)
Fresh yeast extract, 25% aqueous solution (GIBCO/BRL)
Phenol red, 0.1% indicator solution (Fisher)
Penicillin G, 100,000 units/ml
Ultrapure water, 18 ohm, reagent grade, or double-distilled water
NaOH, concentrated solution in utrapure water to adjust pH
NaOH, 1N solution in ultrapure water for minor pH adjustments
HCl, 1N solution in ultrapure water for minor pH adjustments
Petra dishes, sterile, for agar plates
Sterile tubes or bottles for dispensing broth
Autoclave
Water bath, 55°C, for agar only
0.22 μm sterile filtration units
pH meter and calibration buffers
Stir bars and stir plate
Graduated cylinder, sterile, for adding large amounts of serum

PREPARATION

For 200 ml of medium (see discussion below before proceeding):

1. Add these ingredients to ultrapure, endotoxin-free water and mix well.

Mycoplasma broth base	0.7 g
Tryptone	2.0 g
Peptone	1.0 g
Dextrose	1.0 g
Ultrapure water	123.0 ml

   FOR AGAR MEDIUM ONLY
   Agar (SeaPlaque or Noble)   2 g
2. After ingredients are mixed, use concentrated NaOH to adjust pH to 7.5.
3. Autoclave medium at 121°C with 15 pounds pressure (slow exhaust or liquids cycle) for 15 minutes. Allow medium to cool. Medium containing agar should be placed in a 55°C water bath to prevent solidification.
4. Aseptically add:

CMRL-1066 medium	10 ml
Fresh yeast extract	7 ml
Yeastolate	20 ml
Fetal bovine serum	34 ml
Penicillin G	2 ml
Phenol red	4 ml
5. Adjust final pH to 7.5 to 7.6 with sterile 1 N HCl and 1 N NaOH. For broth medium, entire medium may be filter-sterilized after final pH adjustment.

NOTE: The half-life of penicillin in broth or agar is about 7 days at 2–8°C. Therefore, add more penicillin to broth after it has been stored so the concentration of the antimicrobial is high enough to inhibit bacterial growth. If agar plates are to be stored more than 1 week, add twice the amount of penicillin to the medium so there will be enough antibiotic left after 1 week to inhibit bacterial growth. This concentration of penicillin is safe for most mycoplasmas.

6. Store broth and agar at 2–8°C. Broth will remain stable for 1 month at this temperature. Broth may be frozen (−20°C) for 3 months. If there is a precipitate in the medium after freezing, discard the precipitate. (This phenomenon varies among lots of horse serum.)
7. Aseptically dispense broth as needed into sterile tubes and agar into sterile petri dishes. SeaPlaque agarose is a low-gelling-temperature

agarose so agar plates will take longer than usual to solidify at 22–25°C. Agar will not solidify at warmer room temperatures.

8. Medium must be pre-reduced before use by placing it in an aerobic environment. The GasPak anaerobic system from BBL is sufficient for both pre-reduction of the medium and for incubation of cultures.

DISCUSSION

1. Use the manufacturer's instructions for the amount of base (usually given in grams per liter). This amount may vary slightly from lot to lot.

2. Agar preparations can stratify. Be sure the serum and solutions added after autoclaving are well mixed before dispensing final medium. An easy method of mixing is to include a stir bar in the medium before autoclaving, then mix the final medium well, on a stir plate, before dispensing. If the room is very cool, it may be necessary to keep the agar in a 50°C water bath or on a heated stir plate while dispensing.

References

1. Tully JG, Whitcomb RF, Clark HF, Williamson DL: 1977, Pathogenic mycoplasmas: Cultivation and vertebrate pathogenicity of a new spiroplasma. Science 195: 892–894.
2. McGarrity GJ, Rose DL, Kwiastkowski V, Dion AS, Phillips DM, Tully JG. 1983, *Mycoplasma muris* a new species from laboratory mice. Internat J Syst Bacteriol 33: 350–355.

APPENDIX **A8.2.** **Quality Control of all Media**

Each batch of medium must be tested for sterility and for the ability to support the growth of mycoplasmas. Without such testing, negative results are meaningless. If possible, use a relatively fastidious "field strain" of each mycoplasma species of interest as test organisms. Reference mycoplasmal cultures are available from the American Type Culture Collection, Rockville, Maryland, and the National Institutes of Health, NIAID Catalog of Research Reagents, Bethesda, Maryland. We recommend the following stock cultures of the type strains for each species: *M. pulmonis* strain PG34(ASH) (ATCC # 19612); *M. neurolyticum* strain Sabin type A (ATCC #19988); *M. arthritidis* strain Preston (ATCC #19611); *M. collis* strain 58B (ATCC #35278); and *M. muris* strain RIII-4 (ATCC #33757).

Apparently, *M. muris* does not grow on any medium except SP4. Although the other murine mycoplasma species will grow on SP4, they usually grow better with Medium A. Serial dilutions of stock strains of myco-plasmas of known colony-forming units/ml should be used for testing, and the number of organisms that grow in each batch of medium quantified. If the medium does not allow the stock strains to grow to the known concentration, the medium should be discarded.

In addition to quantitive counts of organisms, one also should observe the rate of growth (e.g., how long it takes a culture to grow) and the colonial morphology, as this gives an idea of the ability of the medium to meet the nutritional requirements of the mycoplasmas. One must use a stereomicroscope to view colonies. Some species cannot be seen with the naked eye. When grown on optimal medium, *M. pulmonis* colonies are usually large (easily seen with the naked eye) wet colonies that have little of the typical "fried egg" appearance usually associated with mycoplasmas. The center of the colony is frequently "grainy," and the colonies show little "pitting" of the agar. *M. neurolyticum* and *M. arthritidis* usually do produce "fried egg" colonies. If the medium quality is marginal, the *M. neurolyticum* colonies will be tiny. *M. collis* colonies resemble those of *M. pulmonis,* but do make "fried egg" colonies. *M. muris* colonies tend to be small and granular and seldom the "fried egg" type.

Finally, the appearance of the medium should be inspected. This is usually done as soon as the medium is complete and agar plates have solidified. Broth and agar preparations should be clear and the pH indicator (phenol red), if used, should be the correct color for the desired pH. If agar medium is too hard or too dry, one can usually see microscopic crystals in the medium that resemble calcium oxalate crystals found in urine. Occasionally, a white precipitate forms on the medium or the medium becomes "dry" in appearance. Mycoplasmas usually will not grow on such medium. Cloudy medium is usually due to addition of serum before the medium has cooled sufficiently; cooling to 50°C is sufficient. The serum proteins will denature and precipitate at higher temperatures, resulting in a cloudy solution. Discard any cloudy medium.

Occasionally, one has trouble with inconsistent growth on agar plates made from the same "batch" of medium. In these cases, the trouble is usually traceable to one of two things: use of petri dishes that were sterilized by ethylene oxide rather than irraditation, or incomplete mixing of the final agar medium. As stated in the "Discussion" under media protocols (Appendix A8.1), media containing agar can stratify. If the medium is not mixed well, some plates will not contain all of the nutrients necessary for mycoplasmal growth.

CHAPTER **9**

Canine, Feline, and Equine Mycoplasmas

H. W. WHITFORD
S. W. LINGSWEILER

T he role of mycoplasmas as a cause of disease in dogs, cats, and horses has largely been ignored. Clearly each of these species of mammals harbors mycoplasma organisms, but for the most part, few abnormalities have been associated with them. In some instances, there appears to be the philosophy that since there is an organism present, one must invent a disease to go along with the organism, when, in fact, the data suggest that the mycoplasma is just as common in apparently healthy animals as in diseased animals. Therefore, it is the goal in this section to clarify what is known about mycoplasma infection in dogs, cats, and horses; attempt to place in perspective information that lay publications have spawned; and possibly point out areas of deficiency that would benefit from research efforts.

Canine Mycoplasmas

In 1982, Rosendal reported that 11 species of mycoplasma (*Mycoplasma canis, M. spumans, M. maculosum, M. edwardii, M. cynos, M. molare, M. opalescens, M. feliminutum, M. gateae, M. arginini, M. bovigenitalium*), one unclassified strain, one acholeplasma (*A. laidlawii*), and ureaplasmas of four different serotypes had been isolated from dogs.[9] Doig et al. isolated *M. felis* in addition to eight of the mycoplasmas cited by Rosendal.[1] Mycoplasmas in dogs have been associated with pneumonia, genitourinary tract infections and infertility, colitis and endocarditis. However, mycoplasmas have not been shown to consistently cause any one disease in dogs as a primary pathogen. Rather, they are probably involved as opportunistic organisms, or as one agent in a multifactorial etiology complex. Specific reports of mycoplasma-associated disease conditions in dogs are limited.

Pneumonia

Of five species of mycoplasma recovered from dogs with distemper pneumonia, only *M. cynos* induced a localized pneumonia when endobronchially inoculated into 1-week-old puppies.[8] However, natural cases of pneumonia with *M. cynos* as the sole isolate have not been reported.

Genitourinary Tract Infections and Infertility

Mycoplasmas and ureaplasmas have been recovered from the genitourinary tract of both healthy and diseased dogs, and their specific role has yet to be fully understood. There are, however, some studies that tend to implicate *M. canis* and/or ureaplasmas as having a significant role in genitourinary tract infections and infertility.

Mycoplasmas have been isolated from cystocentesis-collected urine samples in a very small percentage of dogs having suspected urinary tract infections.[9]

The role of *M. canis* and ureaplasmas in genital infections and infertility have been the subject of a couple of studies. *M. canis,* isolated from a bitch with an abnormal estrous cycle, was introduced into the upper genital tract of 4 male dogs and intrauterine into 10 females. Two of the 4 males subsequently developed a chronic orchitis and epididymitis, whereas three of 10 females developed uterine enlargement with histologic evidence of endometritis.[4,6]

Doig et al. cultured for mycoplasmas and ureaplasmas from 136 fertile and infertile, female and male dogs. Mycoplasmas were recovered from 88% of vaginal swabs from females. From males, 85% of preputial swabs and 72% of semen samples were cultured positive. Ureaplasma was found in 50% of females with higher (but not statistically significant) isolations from infertile females, as compared to fertile ones. In males, there was a statistically significant higher number of infertile dogs having both mycoplasmas and ureaplasmas than fertile dogs.[1] The observation was also made from the above report that ureaplasmas were recovered in pure culture from only one male; all other ureaplasma isolations were mixed with mycoplasmas.[7]

A syndrome of infertility, abortion, stillbirths, neonatal deaths, and weak puppies associated with breeding kennels has been described by workers at Cornell.[7] The syndrome may include mucopurulent genital tract discharges in individual animals and should be differentiated from opportunistic bacterial infections. The kennel situation usually favors concentration of organisms, e.g., crowding, intensive management, intermingling of resident and outside animals. Mycoplasmas and/or ureaplasmas, sometimes mixed with bacteria, are recovered from the dams, studs, and aborted or neonatal tissues in all phases of the syndrome.

Isolation of mycoplasmas/ureaplasmas is accomplished by sampling the affected genital tracts (deep vaginal, prepuce, semen) using guarded swabs or any other methods available to reduce bacterial contamination. Samples are then cultured as soon as possible on modified Hayflick's and ureaplasma agar plates, and incubated in broth for subsequent culturing on agar media (see Addendum I). If transporting to lab by commercial carrier, refrigerated shipping in Amies' transport medium without charcoal for mycoplasma (Amies' transport medium w/o charcoal, Difco Laboratories, Detroit, MI) and ureaplasma transport medium for ureaplasma (A3B ureaplasma transport medium, REMEL, Lenexa, KS) should be adequate for preservation. Bacterial cultures may also be made from the Amies' media. Incubation at $35-37°C$ in $5-10\%$ CO_2 with high humidity for up to 10 days resulting in isolation of high numbers of mycoplasmas, ureaplasmas, or mixtures of both along with a clinical history of infertility (with or without active inflammation of the genital tract) should prompt clinicians to give careful consideration to a mycoplasma/ureaplasma-induced infertility syndrome. Bacteria may also be recovered and may be involved as opportunistic pathogens.

Since immunity against mycoplasma does not appear to develop, the affected animals should be separated from healthy kennelmates and treated with appropriate antibiotics (tetracycline or chloramphenicol) until free of the organism. Alternately, individual animals may be neutered and no longer exposed to breeding situations. Additional management changes to reduce concentration of infectious organisms should also be considered.

A popular dog breeding journal article (there may be others) alerted many dog breeders to the realm of mycoplasma.[3] The author of this article reports the facts accurately, but the casual reader is left with the impression that mycoplasmas/ureaplasmas can significantly impair dog reproduction in the United States. Many veterinarians were left out of the information loop, so professional advice to dog breeders was largely unavailable.

Since mycoplasmas/ureaplasmas are common inhabitants of accessible portions of the reproductive tract of healthy fertile dogs, prebreeding cultures may be positive and the pathogenic significance difficult, if not impossible, to interpret. Therefore, prebreeding cultures of healthy dogs have questionable value and should not be encouraged. However, if there is clinical evidence of infertility, sampling for the presence of mycoplasmas and ureaplasmas is highly appropriate, but it is important to consider cultural results relative to other findings. Finally, the clinician must judge whether specific treatment for mycoplasmas/ureaplasmas is likely to solve the infertility problem.

Miscellaneous Canine Conditions Associated with Mycoplasmas

Acholeplasma laidlawii and *M. canis* have been isolated from pericardial sacs of dogs.[5] However, these organisms failed to produce significant pathology in hearts of experimentally inoculated dogs.[2]

At one time, there was speculation that mycoplasmas were involved in the etiology of granulomatous colitis in the Boxer breed.[9] Subsequently, it has been determined that mycoplasmas isolated from the colon are not associated with colitis to any significant extent.

References

1. Doig PA, Ruhnke HL, Bosu WTK: 1981, The genital mycoplasma and ureaplasma flora of healthy and diseased dogs. Can J Comp Med 45:233–238.
2. Eberle G, Kirchhoff H, Amtsberg G, Kersten U, Schütt I, Müller-Peddinghaus R, Trautwein G: 1977, Experimentelle infektion von Hunden mit Trautwein G: 1977, Experimentelle Infektion von Hunden mit Mykoplasmen (*Acholeplasma laidlawii*). Zentrabl Vet (B) 24:689–697.
3. Holum-Hardegen L: Jan 1988, Canine genital mycoplasmosis. Pure-Bred Dogs/American Kennel Gazette, pp. 81–85.
4. Holzmann A, Laber G, Walzl H: 1979, Experimentally induced mycoplasmal infections in the genital tract of the female dog. Theriogenology 12:355–370.
5. Kirchhoff H: 1973, Mykoplasmen bei Hunden. Zentralbl Vet (B) 20:466–473.
6. Laber G, Holzmann A: 1977, Experimentally induced mycoplasmal infection in the genital tract of the male dog. Theriogenology 7:177–188.
7. Lein DH: 1986, Canine mycoplasma, ureaplasma, and bacterial infertility. In: Current Veterinary Therapy IX, ed. Kirk RW, pp. 1240–1243. WB Saunders Co., Philadelphia.
8. Rosendal S: 1978, Canine mycoplasmas: Pathogenicity of mycoplasmas associated with distemper pneumonia. J Infect Dis 138:201–218.
9. Rosendal, S: 1982, Canine mycoplasmas: Their ecologic niche and role in disease. J Am Vet Med Assoc 180:1212–1214.

Feline Mycoplasmas

After reviewing the literature on mycoplasmas in cats, one suspects that surely something has been missed because few reports are found, especially as to the role of mycoplasma in feline disease conditions. In our laboratory experience, we see no indication that mycoplasmas are a problem in cats, in that few, if any, requests are received to specifically look for them in our feline specimens. As of 1979, in a review by Rosendal,[8] only four mycoplasmas (*M. felis, M. gateae, M. feliminutum, M. arginini*), one acholeplasma (*A. laidlawii*) and a ureaplasma were identified as isolates from cats. A more current literature search revealed no additional identified strains. All of the mycoplasma species are recovered from healthy cats. The most common sites for recovery of mycoplasmas are the conjunctiva, nasopharynx, trachea, and urogenital tract.[8]

Only *M. felis* and *M. gateae* have been implicated as having pathogenic significance. *M. felis* has been shown to have a role in feline conjunctivitis and possibly in feline respiratory disease complex.[8,10] Another report links *M. felis* with polyarthritis in an immune-deficient cat.[4] *M. gateae* is usually recovered as a commensal of the upper respiratory and urogenital tract,[8] but some studies indicate that it is a cause of chronic arthritis and tenosynovitis in cats.[3,7] Experimental inoculation of ureaplasma into three pregnant queens resulted in abortion in one queen and a febrile response with neonatal death of offspring in the other two queens.[11]

Unidentified mycoplasmas have been implicated as a cause of abscesses in cats. Mycoplasma was isolated from chronic abscesses in two cats but found not to belong to species *felis, gateae, feliminutum* or *arginini;* specific identification was not possible.[5] These isolates could not be propagated beyond three or four passages, and the possibility of L-form bacteria was never completely ruled out.[9] Another report indicates that an unidentified mycoplasma was involved in a lung abscess in a cat.[2] L-form bacteria have been implicated as a cause of subcutaneous abscesses and arthritis in cats.[1] The etiologic agent was never fully characterized, but L-form seemed most likely due to failure to recover any bacteria or mycoplasma by conventional culture, demonstration of growth of organisms in a special L-form broth, electron microscopic evidence of organisms in affected tissue, and response to tetracycline therapy.

Finally, there is some evidence that mycoplasma may be of zoonotic significance. A veterinarian developed a swollen finger with a discharging sinus following a scratch received from a feline patient he was treating for colitis. *Mycoplasma* sp. as well as *Staphylococcus aureus* was recovered from the discharge and the infection resolved after vibramycin was administered. Prior treatment with staphylococcal-sensitive antibiotics (penicillin, erythromycin, cloxacillin) did not effect a response.[6]

The feline mycoplasmas are not particularly fastidious and should grow using modified Hayflick's medium (see Addendum I) incubated at 37°C in air or with 5–10% CO_2. Acholeplasmas may be recovered at lower temperatures (22–30°C). Swabs of mucosal surfaces directly plated and placed into broth for subsequent plating are usually satisfactory. If tissues are cultured, it is better to push them across plated media rather than

homogenizing them, which tends to release mycoplasmacidal factors.[8]
In summary, mycoplasmas are apparently widespread in the feline host but their specific role as pathogens appears to be limited. Except for conjunctivitis due to *M. felis,* their role may well be influenced by deficiency in the host's defense mechanism, particularly the immunologic system.[8]

References

1. Carro T, Pedersen NC, Beaman BL, Munn R: 1989, Subcutaneous abscesses and arthritis caused by a probable bacterial L-form in cats. J Am Vet Med Assoc 194:1583–1588.
2. Crisp MS, Birchard SJ, Lawrence AE, Fingeroth J: 1987, Pulmonary abscess caused by a *Mycoplasma* sp. in a cat. J Am Vet Med Assoc 191:340–342.
3. Crissman JW: 1986, *Mycoplasma gateae* arthritis in the cat. Dissertation Abstracts International, B. 47:2382.
4. Hooper PT, Ireland LA, Carter A: 1985, Mycoplasma polyarthritis in a cat with probable severe immune deficiency. Aust Vet J 62:352.
5. Keane DP: 1983, Chronic abscesses in cats associated with an organism resembling mycoplasma. Can Vet J 24:289–291.
6. McCabe SJ, Murray JF, Ruhnke HL, Rachlis A: 1987, Mycoplasma infection of the hand acquired from a cat. J Hand Surg 12A:1085–1088.
7. Moise NS, Crissman JW, Fairbrother JF, Baldwin C: 1983, *Mycoplasma gateae* arthritis and tenosynovitis in cats: Case report and experimental reproduction of the disease. Am J Vet Res 44:16–21.
8. Rosendal S: 1979, Canine and feline mycoplasmas. In: The mycoplasmas II, eds. Tully JA, Whitcomb RF, pp. 217–233. Academic Press, New York.
9. Rosendal S: 1990, Personal communication.
10. Tan RJS, Miles JAR: 1974, Incidence and significance of mycoplasma in sick cats. Res Vet Sci 16:27–34.
11. Tan RJS, Miles JAR: 1974, Possible role of feline T-strain mycoplasmas in cat abortion. Aust Vet J 50:142–145.

Equine Mycoplasmas

The mycoplasmas recovered from horses number 17 species: 10 mycoplasmas (*M. equirhinis, M. salivarium, M. arginini, M. subdolum, M. felis, M. equigenitalium, M. pulmonis, M. fastidiosum,* slow glucose metabolizing strains, Strain N3) and 7 Acholeplasmas (*A. laidlawii, A. granularum, A. oculi, A. equifetale, A. hippikon, A. parvum, A.* sp. strain 881).[2,6] These organisms have been recovered from mostly healthy individuals and from specimens collected at slaughterhouses. Isolates were found in the nasopharynx, upper respiratory tract, genitourinary tract and aborted fetal tissues. *Ureaplasma* spp. have not been reported from horses.[2]
The only equine disease condition that has a demonstrated direct causal effect from mycoplasma is pleuritis due to *M. felis.*[3] The organism was isolated in pure culture from pleural fluid of a horse with pleuritis

following treatment with a variety of antibiotics. Experimentally inoculated into a pony, the isolate produced signs of pleuritis, and *M. felis* was recovered at 4 days postinoculation.[3] This experiment was duplicated in 3 additional ponies.[4] In subsequent studies, *M. felis* was found in 3 of 15 horses with pleuritis.[5] An additional 6 of the 15 horses, although culture-negative, had relatively high indirect hemagglutination titers for *M. felis*. Aside from these reports, there is little evidence that *M. felis* pleuritis is a widespread problem in horses. However, it may be involved along with viruses as initiators that allow opportunistic bacteria to become established.[5]

Diagnosis of *M. felis* pleuritis is accomplished by recovering the organism from aspirated pleural fluid collected early in the course of the disease (less than 1 week after onset). The pleural fluid is clarified by centrifugation and the supernatant cultured on Hayflick's medium (see Addendum I). Mycoplasma isolates are identified by indirect immunofluorescence (see Addendum I). Seven days following onset of pleuritis, *M. felis* can no longer be isolated from clinical specimens probably due to presence of antibody against the mycoplasma. Antibody can be detected in the serum using the indirect hemagglutination test.[1]

The other mycoplasmas recovered from horses appear to be commensals (especially acholeplasmas) or possible weak pathogens that require help from other organisms to initiate a disease condition. However, additional studies may reveal that mycoplasmas may play a wider role in equine diseases.

References

1. Cho HJ, Ruhnke HL, Langford EV: 1976, The indirect hemagglutination test for the detection of antibodies in cattle naturally infected with mycoplasmas. Can J Comp Med 40:20–29.
2. Lemke RM: 1979, Equine mycoplasmas. In: The mycoplasmas II, eds. Tully JG, Whitcomb RF, pp. 177–189. Academic Press, New York.
3. Ogilvie TH, Rosendal S, Blackwell TE, Rostkowski CM, Julian RJ, Ruhnke L: 1983, *Mycoplasma felis* as a cause of pleuritis in horses. J Am Vet Med Assoc 182:1374–1376.
4. Rosendal S: 1990, Personal communication.
5. Rosendal S, Blackwell TE, Lumsden JH, Physick-Sheard PW, Viel L, Watson S, Woods P: 1986, Detection of antibodies to *Mycoplasma felis* in horses. J Amer Vet Med Assoc 188:292–294.
6. Tully JG: 1985, Newly discovered mollicutes. In: The mycoplasmas IV, eds. Razin S., Barile MF, pp. 1–26. Academic Press, New York.

A D D E N D A

From the Mycoplasma Workshop
presented at the
5th International Symposium
of the World Association of
Veterinary Laboratory Diagnosticians
Guelph, Ontario, Canada
June 1989

Useful Protocols for Diagnosis of Animal Mycoplasmas

H. L. RUHNKE
Veterinary Laboratory Services
Ontario Ministry of Agriculture and Food
P.O. Box 3612
Guelph, Ontario, Canada N1H 6R8

SØREN ROSENDAL
Veterinary Microbiology and Immunology
Ontario Veterinary College
University of Guelph
Guelph, Ontario, Canada N1G 2W1

ADDENDUM I. Media Formulations and Techniques

Mycoplasma Medium (Hayflick's)[7]

Broth Base
PPLO broth (Difco laboratories, Detroit, MI)	21 g
Distilled, deionized water	1000 ml
Phenol red, 1% solution	2 ml

Adjust pH to 7.4.
Dispense in 500-ml volumes.
Autoclave 121°C 20 minutes
Store 4°C.

Complete Broth
Broth base	75 ml
Unheated horse serum	15 ml
OR Inactivated swine serum	20 ml
Fresh yeast extract, 25% solution	10 ml
Glucose, 50% solution	0.2 ml
Penicillin, 200,000 units/ml	0.5 ml
Thallium acetate, 10% solution	0.2 ml

Complete Agar
PPLO broth powder	1.47 g
Distilled, deionized water	70 ml
Oxoid purified agar	0.8 g

Autoclave 121°C.
Cool to 56°C.
ADD Unheated horse serum	15 ml
OR Inactivated swine serum	20 ml
Fresh yeast extract, 25% solution	10 ml
Glucose, 50% solution	0.2 ml
Penicillin, 200,000 units/ml	0.5 ml
Thallium acetate, 10% solution	0.2 ml

Ureaplasma Medium[11,12]

Broth Base

PPLO broth (Difco)	21 g
Double distilled, deionized water	1000 ml
Phenol red, 1% solution	2 ml

Adjust pH to 6 with 1N HCl.
Dispense 70-ml volumes.
Autoclave 121°C 15 minutes
Store at 4°C.

Complete Broth

Broth base	70 ml
Unheated horse serum	20 ml
Fresh yeast extract, 25% solution	10 ml
Urea, 10% solution	1 ml
Penicillin G potassium, 200,000 units/ml	0.5 ml

Dispense in 3-ml volumes in sterile disposable plastic tubes.
Store at −20°C.

Agar Base

Trypticase Soy broth (BBL, Becton Dickinson, Cockeysville, MD)	2.1 g
Double distilled, deionized water	70 ml
Phenol red, 1% solution	0.2 ml

Adjust pH to 5.5 with 1N HCl.
Oxoid purified agar   0.8 g
Autoclave 121°C 10 minutes
Cool to 56°C.

Complete Agar

Agar base	70 ml
Unheated horse serum	20 ml
Fresh yeast extract, 25% solution	10 ml
Urea, 10% solution	1 ml
Penicillin, 200,000 units/ml	0.5 ml
$MnSO_4$, 3% solution	0.5 ml

Dispense in plates.
Store in closed containers, 4–10°C.
Use within 7–10 days.

Ureaplasma Medium U4 Broth (Buffered)[8]

Hanks' Balanced Salt Solution, 10× concentrate	4 ml
Hartley Digest Broth (Oxoid), **or** Brain heart infusion	
(Difco or Accumedia, Baltimore, MD)	20 ml
Fetal bovine serum	15 ml
Fresh yeast extract, 25% solution	10 ml
Phenol red, 1% solution	0.2 ml
Urea, 10% solution	0.5 ml
Magnesium sulfate, 250 μg/ml	1.0 ml
Penicillin G potassium, 200,000 units/ml	0.5 ml
Double-distilled deionized water to 100 ml	
Buffer: 1.5 M KH_2PO_4 (7 parts)	2.5 ml
1.5 M Na_2HPO_4 (3 parts)	

Fresh Yeast Extract (25%)[6]

Bakers' (Fleischmann's) cake yeast	250 g
Distilled deionized water	1000 ml

Heat to 80°C.
Add yeast while stirring continuously.
Heat to 90–100°C for 5 minutes
Cool. Freeze −20°C
Thaw, centrifuge 1000 G for 45 minutes
Filter supernatant through stacked membrane filters (with nylon mesh separators), 1.2, 0.8, 0.45μ pore size
Dispense in suitable volumes, 10-ml vials
Autoclave at 121°C 2–5 minutes **or** filter sterilize 0.22μ membrane pore size
Store at −20°C up to 3 months

Digitonin Sensitivity[5]

Digitonin	15 mg
Ethanol	0.1 ml

Dispense on blank discs, .025 ml each
Dry overnight at 37°C
Store at 4–10°C
(Stable for several months)

Zone of inhibition: *Mycoplasma* species
No zone of inhibition: *Acholeplasma* species

Controls: for mycoplasma—*M. arginini* or *M. bovis*
        for acholeplasma—*A. laidlawii*

Note: Digitonin is practically insoluble in H_2O; 1 g dissolves in 57 ml absolute alcohol or in 220 ml 95% alcohol.

Fermentation of Glucose

A. PPLO broth   70 ml
   Fresh yeast extract, 25% solution   10 ml
   Inactivated serum, pig or horse   10 ml **or** 20 ml
   Glucose, 50% solution   1 ml
   Penicillin, 200,000 units/ml   0.5 ml
   Phenol red, 1% solution   0.4 ml
B. As above but omit glucose
   Dispense in 5-ml volumes

Method:
   Prepare 24-hour broth culture (10% serum, if it will grow)
   Inoculate approximately 0.05 ml/tube of
      1. broth with glucose
      2. broth without glucose
   Incubate at 37° C
   Subculture after 24 and 48 hrs to confirm growth
   Continue incubation up to 14 days if necessary
   Observe and record any changes in pH; acid (yellow) is positive
   Incubate controls:
      1. uninoculated broth with glucose
      2. uninoculated broth without glucose
   If organism is anaerobic, overlay with 1.5 ml sterile vaseline, paraffin mixture.

Hydrolysis of Arginine

A. PPLO broth, pH = 7.0   70 ml
   Fresh yeast extract, 25% solution   10 ml
   Inactivated serum pig or horse   20 ml
   L-arginine HCl 10% solution   5 ml

Penicillin, 200,000 units/ml	0.5 ml
Phenol red, 1% solution	0.4 ml

B. As above but omit arginine.
Dispense in 5-ml volumes.

Method:
Prepare 24-hour broth culture
Inoculate 0.05 ml/tube of
  1. broth with arginine
  2. broth without arginine
Incubate at 37°C
Subculture to plates after 24 and 48 hours to confirm growth
Continue incubation up to 14 days
Record changes in pH; alkaline (dark red) is positive
Incubate controls:
  1. uninoculated broth with arginine
  2. uninoculated broth without arginine

Phosphatase Activity[4]

PPLO **or** heart infusion broth	74 ml
Purified agar (Oxoid)	0.8 g

Autoclave.
Cool to 56°C.

Inactivated serum, horse **or** swine	20 ml
Fresh yeast extract, 25% solution	10 ml
Sodium phenolphthalein diphosphate, 1% w/v solution	1.0
Penicillin, 200,000 units/ml	0.2 ml

Method:
Inoculate two plates. Inoculate only on one half of each plate either by push block or running drop. Leave the other side uninoculated as a control.

After incubation for 3 and 5 days, test with 5N NaOH. Run a drop across the control side and then the inoculated side. Appearance of a red color in 30 seconds is positive.

If uninoculated side turns red in this time, it means that the serum was not sufficiently inactivated or that the plates are too old.

Positive control: *M. bovis*
Negative control: *M. arginini*

Milk Agar for Casein Hydrolysis[3]

Skim milk powder	32 g
Distilled, deionized water	100 ml

Sterilize 10 minutes 112–115°C
Prepare Hayflick's agar with 20% HS, 10% yeast etc.
Cool to 56°C
Add 1 part skim milk to 7 parts medium
Pour plates

Positive control: *M. mycoides* subsp. *mycoides,* LC-type, e.g., strain
Y3343; positive reaction is a clear zone around colonies.
Negative control: *M. alkalescens*

Indirect Fluorescent Antibody Test (FA)[1,10]

1. You need colonies small and close together, but separated. Large colonies sometimes give equivocal results.
2. Plates ready for FA can be kept in the refrigerator for 2–4 weeks in plastic bags or boxes to keep them from drying out.
3. Cut strips of agar that contain colonies and place on microscope slide. Cut strips into approximately 5 mm squares. Place the blocks far enough apart so that the sera will not run together.
4. Fix to the slide by embedding squares in a mixture of 65% paraffin and 35% Vaseline.[1] Six to eight squares can be placed on one slide (the wax should not be higher than the agar).
5. Place a drop of buffer on each square while you prepare the antiserum dilutions. This helps to rehydrate the agar so the blocks will not absorb too much serum.
6. Prepare serum dilutions in buffer, pH 7.2–7.4. Do not use serum undiluted or 1/10; you may get false negatives.
7. Remove excess buffer from surface of each block with tissue. Do not blot the top surface.
8. Place one drop of diluted antiserum on each block.
9. Incubate at room temperature 30 minutes in moist chamber.
10. Wash 2 × 10 minutes in phosphate buffer.

11. Remove excess buffer from each block.
12. Place one drop of fluorescein-conjugated anti-rabbit globulin on each block.
13. Predetermine the dilution of each batch of conjugate, usually 1/20 or 1/30.
14. Incubate at room temperature 30 minutes in moist chamber.
15. Wash 2 × 10 minutes in phosphate buffer.
16. Read with epi-fluorescent illumination.

This method allows you to identify more than one species when the culture is mixed. Stained blocks can be stored at 4–10°C in a moist chamber for several days if desired.

Precipitation of Serum for Indirect FA

5 ml saturated $(NH_4)_2SO_4$
10 ml serum — add slowly, drop-wise, to $(NH_4)_2SO_4$ with continuous stirring; stir overnight at 4°C
Centrifuge at 6000 rpm, 10 minutes, 4–10°C (Sorvall)
Resuspend precipitate in 10 ml distilled water
Add to 5 ml $(NH_4)_2SO_4$ as above
Stir 1½ hrs at room temperature
Centrifuge at 6000 rpm, 10 minutes, 4–10°C
Resuspend in 3.3 ml distilled water
Dialyze overnight with saline
Measure volume and bring up to original volume with PBS, pH 7.5
Store −20°C
Use for indirect FA method

Precipitated serum reduces background staining in the indirect method.

Conjugation of Serum with Fluorescein Isothiocyanate (FITC)

1. Precipitate globulin by ⅓ saturation with ammonium sulfate; e.g., add drop-wise 10 ml serum to 5 ml saturated ammonium sulfate with continuous stirring. Stir overnight at 4°C.
2. Centrifuge at 6000 rpm, 10 minutes, 4–10°C (Sorvall).
3. Redissolve precipitate in distilled water equal to ⅓ of original serum volume.
4. Dialyze against saline at 4°C with stirring. Change saline 3–4 times during day and continue dialysis overnight.
5. Remove from casing and measure volume.

6. Add PBS pH 7.5 to bring total volume to twice the original serum volume.
7. Determine protein content of solution by spectrophotometer at 280 nm.

$$\frac{O.D.}{13.7} \times \text{dilution factor} \times 10 = \text{mg protein/ml}$$

$$\times \text{vol.} = \text{total protein}$$

8. Prepare fresh carbonate-bicarbonate buffer:

0.5 M pH 9.0
Sodium bicarbonate $NaHCO_3$, 0.37 g
Sodium carbonate $NaCO_3$, 0.06 g

Dissolve and bring to 10 ml with distilled water
9. Add carbonate-bicarbonate buffer to protein solution in a ratio of 1:1.
10. Weigh FITC in an amount equal to 1/60 of the total protein.
11. Dissolve FITC in small volume carbonate-bicarbonate buffer.
12. Add drop by drop VERY SLOWLY to protein solution on stirrer.
13. React overnight at 4°C with continuous stirring, or 3 hours at room temperature.
14. Prepare Sephadex G25 or G50 column, 12 mm diameter.

Pack to height of 3.5 cm/ml of serum to be used.
Equilibrate and run with Tris-HCl buffer 0.1M pH 8.7.

15. Apply protein-FITC solution to column.
Elute with Tris-HCl pH 8.7 and collect first peak.
(Steps 16 and 17 are optional.)
16. Apply this fraction to a DEAE-cellulose column equilibrated with Tris-HCl buffer.
Adjust flow rate to 0.7–1.0 ml/minute
Elute with Tris-HCl 0.1M pH 8.7,
then Tris-HCl 0.1M pH 8.7 + 0.1M NaCl
then Tris-HCl 0.1M pH 8.7 + 0.2M NaCl
17. Concentrate fractions if necessary.
18. Test conjugate with homologous organism.
19. Store in small volumes in sealed ampules in −70°C.

Tris-HCl Buffer 0.1M pH 8.7
Tris hydroxymethyl aminomethane M.W. = 121.4

Dissolve 48.46 g in distilled water
Bring to 3990 ml
Adjust pH to 8.7 with HCl
Bring volume to 4000 ml

Antigen Preparation for Immunization

1. For mycoplasmas: Prepare 500–1000 ml broth. Use 1% serum fraction or 20% rabbit serum in place of horse serum.
   For ureaplasmas: Prepare 1000 ml Howard's U4 broth with 2.5% buffer.
2. Centrifuge broth at 15,000 g for 1 hour
   Filter through 0.22 μm membrane filter to sterilize.
3. Inoculate with culture. Incubate appropriate time.
4. Centrifuge 15,000 g, 4°C, 1 hour.
   Wash sediment twice in PBS pH 7.2–7.5.
5. For mycoplasmas, resuspend sediment in 15–20 ml PBS.
   For ureaplasmas, resuspend in 10 ml.
   Plate on mycoplasma or ureaplasma agar to check growth.
   Plate drops on blood agar to check purity.
6. Store in 1 ml volumes at −70°C.

Rabbit Immunization Procedure for Mycoplasmas/ Ureaplasmas

Immunization Schedule
   Pre-bleed and test serum:
      for mycoplasmas — by growth inhibition and FA
      for ureaplasmas — by metabolic inhibition and FA
Day 0
   Emulsify 2 ml antigen suspension with 2 ml Freund's complete adjuvant.
   Emulsion is ready when a drop on the surface of water does not spread but remains intact.
   Amount recovered from this mixture is usually about 3 ml.
   Inject 0.2 ml sub-Q into 8 sites along back.
   Inject 0.5 ml intramuscularly into each hip.
Day 21
   Inject 1 ml antigen (without adjuvant) intravenously 3 times per week for 6 injections.

OR

Repeat schedule for day 0.

Day 40

   Test blood.

   Test for growth or metabolic inhibition and FA.

Day 43

   If serum satisfactory, bleed rabbit out.

   If serum unsatisfactory repeat IV injections, as on day 21.

OR

   Give a single 3-ml dose IV.

   Test-bleed 7 days after last injection.

   Bleed out no later than 10 days after last injection.

   If serum is still unsatisfactory, it is probably best to immunize another
     rabbit.

Semen Culture[13]

A. Raw Semen
   1. Plate 2 × 0.01 ml drops of undiluted semen onto:
      a) mycoplasma (Hayflick's) agar with porcine serum
      b) ureaplasma agar.
   2. Make 4 10-fold dilutions in ureaplasma broth.
   3. Make 4 dilutions in Hayflick's broth with porcine serum.
   4. Plate 2 × 0.01 ml drops of 10^{-1} dilutions onto corresponding
      plates.
   5. Subculture from broth to plates on day 2, and again on day 4 (or
      5).
   6. Incubate plates for 10 days before discarding as negative.
      Incubate broths aerobically.
      Incubate mycoplasma plates in 5–7% CO_2.
      Incubate ureaplasma plates anaerobically (we use the H_2 + CO_2
      system).
   7. Observe ureaplasma broths daily for color change, and subculture
      to agar as soon as color changes to light pink.
   8. Read plates every 2 days for mycoplasma and ureaplasma colonies.
   9. Incubate plates for 10 days before discarding as negative.

We always confirm a color change in ureaplasma broth by subculture to
agar. Some arginine hydrolyzing mycoplasmas and some diphtheroids can
cause a color change without turbidity.

B. Processed Semen
   1. Surface-sterilize semen straw with a cotton gauze soaked in 70%
      alcohol and let air dry.

2. Aseptically remove semen from straw and place in sterile tube.
3. Plate 2 × 0.01-ml drops undiluted semen onto:
   a) mycoplasma (Hayflick's) agar with porcine serum
   b) ureaplasma agar.
4. Make ¹⁄₁₀ dilution in mycoplasma broth base (without serum or yeast). PBS is used by some but can be inhibitory after 1 hour exposure.
   a) plate 2 × 0.01-ml drops onto mycoplasma agar.
   b) plate 2 × 0.01-ml drops onto ureaplasma agar.
5. Centrifuge 35,000 × G, 20 minutes, 4–10°C.
6. Resuspend sediment in 10 ml broth base.
7. Centrifuge 35,000 × G, 20 minutes, 4–10°C.
8. Repeat steps 6 and 7.
9. Discard supernatant.
10. Resuspend sediment in 1 ml broth base.
11. Plate 2 × 0.01-ml running drops to mycoplasma plate.
12. Plate 2 × 0.01-ml running drops to ureaplasma plate.
13. Make 4 10-fold dilutions in ureaplasma broth.
14. Make one 10-fold dilution in mycoplasma broth.
15. Incubate all broths aerobically.
    Incubate mycoplasma plates in 5–7% CO_2.
    Incubate ureaplasma plates anaerobically.
16. Observe ureaplasma broths daily for color change, and subculture to agar as soon as color changes to light pink.
17. Read plates every 2 days for mycoplasma and ureaplasma colonies.
18. Subculture mycoplasma broth to plates at 2 and 4 (or 5) days.
19. Incubate plates for 10 days before discarding as negative.

Passive Hemagglutination Test

1. **Phosphate-buffered glucose (PBG)**

Disodium phosphate 0.15M	76 ml
Monopotassium phosphate 0.15M	24 ml
Glucose 5.4% in distilled water	100 ml

pH should be 7.2.

Store in refrigerator.

2. **Red blood cells**
   Collect sheep blood in Alsever's solution.
   Wash 4 times in PBG, 2000 × g, 4°C, 10 minutes each.
   Make 20% suspension in PBG.

3. a) **Glutaraldehyde 0.2%**

Glutaraldehyde (EM) 25% aqueous solution   0.8 ml

PBG   99.2 ml

b) **Glutaraldehyde-fixed red cells**

Mix equal volumes:

20% sheep cell suspension

0.2% glutaraldehyde

Incubate in 37°C water bath, 15 minutes mix occasionally.

Wash 5 times with 0.85% saline, 450 × G, 5°C, 10 minutes.

Make a 10% suspension in saline.

Add sodium azide to make 0.1% final concentration.

4. **Mycoplasma antigen**

Grow mycoplasmas in appropriate medium 2–3 days depending on rate of growth.

Centrifuge 14,000 × G, 1 hour, 5°C.

Wash twice with saline – 14,000 × G, 30 minutes, 5°C.

Resuspend in saline, 5 ml/L of culture.

Reserve 0.5 ml for protein determination.

Store frozen at −70°C.

Determine protein concentration by Lowry[9] method or Bradford[2] method (BioRad protein assay, BioRad Chemical Division, Richmond, CA).

Adjust volume to make a suspension of 10 mg protein/ml.

5. **Sensitization of glutaraldehyde-fixed red cells with mycoplasma antigen**

Centrifuge glutaraldehyde-fixed cells, 450 × G, 10 minutes 5°C.

Wash twice with 0.01M PBS, same speed and time.

Make a 20% suspension in PBS.

To 5 ml of the 20% glutaraldehyde-fixed cells, add 2 ml antigen adjusted to 10 mg protein/ml.

Add sodium azide to make a final concentration of 0.1%.

Mix thoroughly.

Incubate 37°C overnight (16–18 hrs) with occasional agitation.

Centrifuge 450 × G, 10 minutes, 5°C.

Wash 3 times in PBS same speed and time.

Resuspend at 2% concentration in PBS.

Store at 5°C.

References

1. Al-Aubaidi JM, Fabricant J: 1971, The practical application of immunofluorescence (agar block technic) for the identification of mycoplasma. Cornell Vet 61:519–542.

2. Bradford MM: 1976, A rapid and sensitive method for the quantitation of microgram quantities of protein utilizing the principle of protein-dye binding. Anal biochem 72:248–254.

3. Cottew GS, Yeats FR: 1978, Subdivision of *Mycoplasma mycoides* subsp. *mycoides* from cattle and goats into two types. Austral Vet J 54: 293–296.

4. Ernø H, Stipkovits L: 1973, Bovine mycoplasmas: Cultural and biochemical studies II. Acta Vet Scand 14:450–463.

5. Freundt EA, Andrews BE, Ernø H, Kunze M, Black FT: 1973, The sensitivity of Mycoplasmatales to sodium-polyanethol-sulfate and digitonin. Zbl Bakt I, Abt Orig A 225:104–112.

6. Friis NF: 1975, Some recommendations concerning primary isolation of *Mycoplasma suipneumoniae* and *Mycoplasma flocculare*. Nord Vet Med 27: 337–339.

7. Hayflick L: 1965, Tissue cultures and mycoplasmas. Texas Reports on Biology and Medicine 23:285–303.

8. Howard CJ, Gourlay RN, Collins J: 1978, Serological studies with bovine ureaplasmas. Int J Syst Bact 28:473–477.

9. Lowry OH, Rosebrough NJ, Farr AL, Randall RJ: 1951, Protein measurement with the Folin phenol reagent. J Biol Chem 193:265–275.

10. Rosendal S, Black FT: 1972, Direct and indirect immunofluorescence of unfixed and fixed mycoplasma colonies. Acta Path Microbiol Scand 80-B:615–622.

11. Shepard MC: 1969, Fundamental biology of the T-strains. In Hayflick L (ed) The Mycoplasmatales, pp. 49–65. Appleton-Century-Crofts, New York.

12. Shepard MC: 1976, Differential agar medium (A7) for identification of *Ureaplasma urealyticum* (Human T mycoplasmas) in primary cultures of clinical material. J Clin Microbiol 3:613–625.

13. Truscott RB, Ruhnke HL: 1984, Control of *Mycoplasma* and *Ureaplasma* in semen. In Stalheim OHV (ed), Proc Int Symp on Microbiological Tests for the International Exchange of Animal Genetic Material, pp. 50–65. Am Assoc Vet lab Diagn Suppl.

ADDENDUM **II. Protocol for Animal Mycoplasmas**

MYCOPLASMA AGAR
Horse & Swine Serum
CO_2

Colonies

NEGATIVE REPORT
after 10 days

POSITIVE

UREAPLASMA AGAR

Anaerobic

Colonies

NEGATIVE REPORT
after 7 days

brown

UREAPLASMA

Epi-immunofluorescence on colonies on agar

NEGATIVE

Biochemicals
    Digitonin, glucose,
        arginine, phosphatase
        casein

Epi-immunofluorescence

POSITIVE

MYCOPLASMA SPECIES

>80 species

MYCOPLASMA BROTH
Horse and Swine Serum

Aerobic

SUBCULTURE TO AGAR

156

2-3 days

CO_2

4-7 days

Colonies

POSITIVE

NEGATIVE

UREAPLASMA BROTH

$10^{-1 \ to \ -4}$

Aerobic

Alkaline

No change after 7 days
NEGATIVE

SUBCULTURE TO AGAR

Anaerobic

Ureaplasma agar
w $MnSO_4$

Brown colonies

UREAPLASMA

U4 agar

Colorless colonies

FA for serotype
on bovine isolates

Glucose positive, arginine negative mycoplasmas

Phosphatase negative:

M. bovirhinis
M. bovoculi
M. canis
M. capricolum
M. columborale
M. conjunctivae
M. dispar
M. edwardii
M. fastidiosum
M. feliminutum
M. flocculare
M. gallinaceum
M. gallisepticum
M. gallopavonis
M. hyopneumoniae
M. molare
M. mycoides subsp. *mycoides*
M. mycoides subsp. *capri*
M. neurolyticum
M. ovipneumoniae
M. pneumoniae
M. pullorum
M. pulmonis
M. synoviae
Bovine serogroup 7 (try possibly
   serogroup L)
Caprine/ovine serogroup 6
Caprine/ovine serogroup 8
F38

Phosphatase positive:

M. anatis
M. capricolum
M. caviae
M. citelli
M. cynos
M. equigenitalium
M. felis

M. hyorhinis (sometimes false glu-
cose negative)
M. putrefaciens
HRC689
Caprine/ovine serogroup 6
M. mustelae

Glucose positive, arginine positive mycoplasmas

Phosphatase negative:

M. alvi
M. fermentans
M. iowae (try possibly also avian
group J,K,N,Q, or R)
M. sualvi
Caprine/ovine serogroup 6

Phosphatase positive:

M. alvi
M. capricolum
M. caviae
M. fermentans
M. moatsii
M. sualvi
Caprine/ovine serogroup 6

Glucose negative, arginine positive mycoplasmas

Phosphatase negative:

M. arginini
M. canadense
M. columbinum
M. equirhinis
M. faucium
M. gallinarum
M. gateae
M. hominis
M. hyosynoviae
M. iners
M. lipophilum
M. orale
M. salivarium
M. subdolum

Phosphatase positive:

M. alkalescens
M. arthritidis
M. buccale
M. columbinasale
M. hyopharyngis
M. lipophilum
M. maculosum
M. meleagridis
M. opalescens
M. primatum
M. spumans
M. subdolum
Caprine/ovine serogroup 5
694

Glucose negative, arginine negative mycoplasmas

Phosphatase negative:

M. bovigenitalium
M. feliminutum
Caprine/ovine group 7

Phosphatase positive:

M. agalactiae
M. bovigenitalium
M. bovis
M. californicum
M. citelli
M. verecundum
Caprine/ovine serogroup 11

Avian Mycoplasmas

Mycoplasmas:

M. anatis
M. columbinasale
M. columbinum
M. columborale
M. gallinaceum
M. gallinarum
M. gallisepticum
M. gallopavonis
M. iners

	M. iowae
	M. meleagridis
	M. pullorum
	M. synoviae

Acholeplasmas: *A. axanthum*
1. Glucose positive, arginine positive:
   a. phosphatase negative: *M. iowae*
2. Glucose negative, arginine positive:
   a. phosphatase negative: *M. columbinum*
                         M. gallinarum
                         M. iners
   b. phosphatase positive: *M. columbinasale*
                         M. meleagridis
3. Glucose positive, arginine negative:
   a. phosphatase negative: *M. columborale*
                         M. gallinaceum
                         M. gallisepticum
                         M. gallopavonis
                         M. pullorum
                         M. synoviae
   b. phosphatase positive: *M. anatis*
4. Glucose negative, arginine negative   none

Bovine Mycoplasmas

Mycoplasmas: *M. alkalescens*
                         M. alvi
                         M. arginini
                         M. bovigenitalium
                         M. bovirhinis
                         M. bovis
                         M. bovoculi
                         M. californicum
                         M. canadense
                         M. conjunctivae
                         M. dispar

M. equirhinis
M. gallinarum
M. gallisepticum
M. gateae
M. mycoides subsp. *mycoides*
M. verecundum
Group 7 (PG50) (*Leach)

Acholeplasmas:

1. Glucose positive, arginine positive:
    a. phosphatase negative:
    b. phosphatase positive:
2. Glucose negative, arginine positive:
    a. phosphatase negative:

    b. phosphatase positive:

3. Glucose positive, arginine negative:
    a. phosphatase negative:

4. Glucose negative, arginine negative:
    a. phosphatase negative:
    b. phosphatase positive:

A. axanthum
A. laidlawii
A. modicum

M. alvi
M. alvi

M. arginini
M. canadense
M. equirhinis
M. gallinarum
M. gateae
M. alkalescens
M. canadense

M. bovirhinis
M. bovoculi
M. conjunctivae
M. dispar
M. gallisepticum
M. mycoides subsp. *mycoides*
Group 7 (PG50)

M. bovigenitalium
M. bovigenitalium
M. bovis
M. californicum
M. verecundum

Canine and Feline Mycoplasmas

Mycoplasmas (dogs):

M. arginini
M. bovigenitalium
M. canis
M. cynos
M. edwardii
M. feliminutum
M. felis
M. gateae
M. maculosum
M. molare
M. opalescens
M. spumans
HRC689

Acholeplasma (dogs and cats):

A. laidlawii

Mycoplasmas (cats):

M. arginini
M. feliminutum
M. gateae

1. Glucose positive, arginine
   positive: none
2. Glucose negative, arginine
   positive:
   a. phosphatase negative: *M. arginini*
                                     M. gateae
   b. phosphatase positive: *M. maculosum*
                                     M. opalescens
                                     M. spumans

3. Glucose positive, arginine
   negative:
   a. phosphatase negative: *M. canis*
                                     M. edwardii
                                     M. feliminutum
                                     M. molare
   b. phosphatase positive: *M. cynos*
                                     M. felis
                                     HRC689

4. Glucose negative, arginine
   negative:
   a. phosphatase negative: *M. bovigenitalium*
                                     M. feliminutum
   b. phosphatase positive: *M. bovigenitalium*

Equine Mycoplasmas

Mycoplasmas:	*M. arginini**
	M. bovigenitalium*
	M. equigenitalium
	M. equirhinis
	M. fastidiosum
	M. feliminutum*
	M. felis (related)
	M. mycoides (related)*
	M. pulmonis (related)*
	M. salivarium*
	M. subdolum
Acholeplasmas:	*A. axanthum**
	A. equifetale
	A. granularum*
	A. hippikon
	A. laidlawii
	A. modicum
	A. oculi

1. Glucose positive, arginine positive: none
2. Glucose negative, arginine positive:
   a. phosphatase negative: *M. arginini*
      M. equirhinis
      M. salivarium
      M. subdolum
   b. phosphatase positive: *M. subdolum*
3. Glucose positive, arginine negative:
   a. phosphatase negative: *M. fastidiosum*
      M. feliminutum
      M. mycoides (related)
      M. pulmonis (related)
   b. phosphatase positive: *M. equigenitalium*
      M. felis (related)
4. Glucose negative, arginine negative:
   a. phosphatase negative: *M. bovigenitalium*
      M. feliminutum
   b. phosphatase positive: *M. bovigenitalium*

*Occasional isolates only.

Caprine and Ovine Mycoplasmas

Mycoplasmas:	*M. agalactiae*
	M. arginini
	M. bovis
	M. capricolum
	M. conjunctivae
	M. gallinarum
	M. mycoides subsp. *capri*
	M. mycoides subsp. *mycoides*
	M. ovipneumoniae
	M. putrefaciens
	F38-like group
	Group 5 (Goat 145)
	Group 6 (Goat 189)
	Group 7 (A 1343)
	Group 8 (Y-goat)
	Group 11 (2-D)
Acholeplasmas:	*A. granularum*
	A. laidlawii
	A. oculi

The grouping system is according to Al-Aubaidi.

1. Glucose positive, arginine
   positive:
   a. phosphatase negative: Group 6 (Goat 189)
   b. phosphatase positive: *M. capricolum*
2. Glucose negative, arginine
   positive:
   a. phosphatase negative: *M. arginini*
                                  M. gallinarum
   b. phosphatase positive: Group 5 (Goat 145)
3. Glucose positive, arginine
   negative:
   a. phosphatase negative: *M. capricolum*
                                  M. conjunctivae
                                  M. mycoides subsp. *capri*
                                  M. mycoides subsp. *mycoides*
                                  M. ovipneumoniae
                                  Group 6 (Goat 189)
                                  Group 8 (Y-goat)
                                  F38-like group (F38; C758)
   b. phosphatase positive: *M. capricolum*
                                  M. putrefaciens

4. Glucose negative, arginine
   negative:
   a. phosphatase negative: Group 7 (A1343)
   b. phosphatase positive: *M. agalactiae*
                                   M. bovis
                                   Group 11 (2-D)

Porcine Mycoplasmas

Mycoplasmas: *M. arginini**
                                   M. bovigenitalium*
                                   M. buccale*
                                   M. flocculare
                                   M. hyopharyngis
                                   M. hyopneumoniae
                                   M. hyorhinis
                                   M. hyosynoviae
                                   M. sualvi
Acholeplasmas: *A. axanthum**
                                   A. granularum*
                                   A. laidlawii
                                   A. modicum*
                                   A. oculi*

1. Glucose positive, arginine
   positive:
   a. phosphatase negative: *M. sualvi*
   b. phosphatase positive: *M. sualvi*
2. Glucose negative, arginine
   positive:
   a. phosphatase negative: *M. arginini*
   b. phosphatase positive: *M. buccale*
                                   M. hyopharyngis (film)

3. Glucose positive, arginine
   negative:
   a. phosphatase negative: *M. flocculare*
                                   M. hyopneumoniae
   b. phosphatase positive: *M. hyorhinis* (sometimes
                                   false glucose negative)

4. Glucose negative, arginine
   negative:
   b. phosphatase positive: *M. bovigenitalium*
*Occasional isolates only.

Index